T0225742

Single Point Acupuncture and Moxibustion For 100 Diseases

(Second Edition)

Written By,
Dr. Decheng Chen
Ph.D. L.Ac.

Edited by: Erin Hessel

Order this book online at www.trafford.com
or email orders@trafford.com

Most Trafford titles are also available at major online book retailers.

The information, ideas, and suggestions in this book are not intended as a substitute
for professional medical advice. Before following any suggestions contained in this
book, you should consult your personal physician. Neither the author nor the publisher
shall be liable or responsible for any loss or damage allegedly arising as a consequence
of your use or application of any information or suggestions in this book.

Printed in the United States of America.

ISBN: 978-1-4269-3721-7 (sc)
ISBN: 978-1-4269-3722-4 (e)

Library of Congress Control Number: 2010910307

*Our mission is to efficiently provide the world's finest, most comprehensive book publishing
service, enabling every author to experience success. To find out how to publish your book,
your way, and have it available worldwide, visit us online at www.trafford.com*

Trafford rev. 09/09/2010

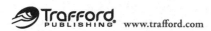 www.trafford.com

North America & international
toll-free: 1 888 232 4444 (USA & Canada)
phone: 250 383 6864 ♦ fax: 812 355 4082

Preface

Chinese Acupuncture and Moxibustion have had a long history. The practice of Single Point Acupuncture and Moxibustion Therapy occupies a special place in this field. This is the first book published on this particular technique.

Single Point Acupuncture and Moxibustion for 100 Diseases offers a thorough description of the clinical application of single point acupuncture and moxibustion. Single point acupuncture and moxibustion therapy are defined by selecting one point during each acupuncture session for the treatment and prevention of specific ailments. The single point technique is noted for its fewer point selection treatments, quick therapeutic response, and exceptional results. It is a simple protocol for practitioners to use and readily accepted by patients.

The Chinese version of this book, which I wrote and published in 1998 and is very popular amongst readers across the world, is entitled ***The Chinese Single Point Acupuncture and Moxibustion.*** From this original book, 100 diseases were chosen to be translated and published into English as the first version in 2000.

Since the first edition in English, ***Single Point Acupuncture and Moxibustion for 100 Diseases*** has been updated to include the most proven and efficient point-prescriptions and applications for medical doctors and acupuncturists to use in their practice. Proven treatments from the previous book are combined with more than twenty years of clinical experience provide excellent results and valuable information in this newer edition.

This book consists of five chapters: Painful Diseases; Internal Medicine; Surgical Applications; Obstetrics, Gynecology and Pediatrics; and Ophthalmic, Ear, Nose and Throat Ailments. Within these sections are included approximately 100 specific and common clinical ailments. Some of the pathologies include headache, neck pain, sciatica, abdominal pain, arrhythmia, hypertension, common cold, bronchitis, irregular menstruation, bronchial-asthma in children, infantile diarrhea, eczema, urticaria, tinnitus, deafness, toothache, smoking cessation, and weight loss. All of the disorders covered in this book are listed by their western medical disease names, most of which are explained in both western medical and traditional Chinese medicine theories. Every chapter of this book is consistent with a simple and clear style and format. Each section consists of an introduction to the disease, the one point selected, detailed needle technique explanation, proven efficacy, case study of the treatment, and discussion.

This edition puts a special emphasis on the acupuncture method and needle techniques. When applying the suggested prescriptions in clinical practice, the instructions should be followed step by step in the easy-to-use format of this book. In this way, the practitioner can expect to receive the same results that are mentioned in the book.

These applications are not only for acupuncturists in the United States, but for medical doctors and acupuncturists around the world. This book includes methods and techniques such as acupuncture, electro-acupuncture, moxibustion, cupping therapy, three-edged needle therapy, intradermal needle therapy, cutting therapy, embedding therapy and point injection therapy. The practitioner must take careful note of laws and regulations in their area and practice according to what is legal in their State or Country.

Finally, I wish to thank Mr. Ying Che Huang and Ms. Chien Huei Lin for the new cover design.

The author: Dr. Decheng Chen

January 30, 2010, New York

Contents

Preface v

Chapter I Painful Diseases 1

1.1 Headache 1

1.2 Pain of the Supraorbital Area 3

1.3 Migraine 4

1.4 Trigeminal Neuralgia 6

1.5 Occipital Neuralgia 7

1.6 Stiff Neck 8

1.7 Cervical Spondylopathy 10

1.8 Periarthritis of the Shoulder 12

1.9 Brachialgia 14

1.10 Tennis Elbow 15

1.11 Wrist and Ankle Sprain 16

1.12 Shoulder and Back Pain 17

1.13. Intercostal Neuralgia 19

1.14 Lumbar Transverse Process Syndrome 20

1.15 Acute Lumbar Muscle Sprain 21

1.16 Chronic Lumbar Muscle Strain 23

1.17 Sciatica 25

1.18 Pain in Lower Back and Leg. 27

1.19 Heel Pain 28

1.20 Knee pain. 29

1.21 General pain. 31

1.22 Angina Pectoris 32

1.23 Cholecystalgia 33

1.24 Renal colic 35

1.25 Gastrospasm. 36

1.26 Acute Abdominal Pain 37

1.27 Toothache. 39

Chapter II Internal Diseases **42**

2.1 Arrhythmia 42

2.2 Coronary Atherosclerotic Cardiopathy. 43

2.3 Hypertension 44

2.4 Hypotension 45

2.5 Common Cold. 46

2.6 Bronchitis. 48

2.7 Bronchial Asthma. 49

2.8 Hiccup. 52

2.9 Chronic Gastritis 53

2.10 Vomiting 54

2.11 Diarrhea. 56

2.12 Constipation 57

2.13 Retention of Urine 59

2.14 Urinary Incontinence. 60

2.15 Impotence 62

2.16 Seminal Emission. 63

2.17 Facial Paralysis 64

2.18 Facial Spasm. 65

2.19 Sequelae to Cerebrovascular Accident. 66

2.20 Rheumatic Chorea 68

2.21 Spasmodic Torticollis 70

2.22 Numbness of the Hand 71

2.23 Systremma 72

2.24 Epilepsy 73

2.25 Vertigo. 74

2.26 Schizophrenia. 75

2.27 Hysteria 76

2.28 Insomnia 78

Chapter III Surgical Diseases. 80

3.1 Chronic Cholecystitis. 80

3.2 Cholelithiasis 81

3.3 Biliary Ascariasis. 82

3.4 Volvulus. 83

3.5 Acute Mastitis 84

3.6 Ureterolithiasis. 85

3.7 Chronic Prostatitis 85

3.8 Hemorrhoids 86

3.9 Eczema. 88

3.10 Urticaria. 89

3.11 Cutaneous Pruritus. 90

3.12 Psoriasis 91

3.13 Acne. 92

3.14 Vitiligo. 93

Chapter IV Obstetrical, Gynecological and Pediatric Diseases 94

    4.1 Dysfunctional Uterine Bleeding 94

    4.2 Dysmenorrhea 96

    4.3 Leukorrhagia 97

    4.4 Infertility 99

    4.5 Pelvic Inflammatory Disease 100

    4.6 Morning sickness 101

    4.7 Abnormal Position of the Fetus 102

    4.8 Prolonged or Difficult Labor 103

    4.9 Postpartum Retention of Urine 104

    4.10 Postpartum Complications 105

    4.11 Hypogalactia (Insufficient Lactation) 106

    4.12 Childhood Mumps 107

    4.13 Infantile Diarrhea 108

    4.14 Enuresis 109

    4.15 Excessive Night Crying 111

Chapter V: Ophthalmic, Ear-Nose-Throat Diseases and Others 112

    5.1 Hordeolum 112

    5.2 Lacrimation (Tearing) 113

    5.3 Optic Atrophy 114

    5.4 Myopia 116

    5.5 Deafness 117

    5.6 Tinnitus 118

    5.7 Meniere's disease 119

    5.8 Rhinitis 120

    5.9 Epistaxis 121

    5.10 Acute Tonsillitis 122

5.11 Plum-Pit Qi of the Throat 123

5.12 Oral Ulcerations. 124

5. 13 TMJ Syndrome 124

5.14 Smoking Cessation 125

5.15 Dispelling the Effects of Alcohol 127

5.16 Weight Loss 127

About the Author 129

The Author's Publishing List 130

Chapter I Painful Diseases

1.1 Headache

Headache is a subjective symptom that occurs for a variety of reasons and accompanies many acute and chronic diseases. The type of headache discussed in this chapter refers to the "headache" as the main symptom present, regardless of etiology or other disorders. For example, a headache may be seen with infectious febrile diseases, hypertension, intracranial disease, traumatic injury, psychoneurosis, migraine, and others.

Point

Fengchi (GB 20)

Location

Fengchi (GB 20) is located on the nape of the neck, below the occipital bone, on the level of Fengfu (DU 16), and in the depression between the heads of the sternocloidomastoid and trapezius muscles.

Methods

1. Acupressure is used. With the patient in a seated position, use the thumb and middle finger of the right hand to squeeze Fengchi (GB 20) on both sides using pressure and/or rolling technique. Begin in this manner on both sides first mildly, then gradually increasing in intensity. For one course of treatment, this procedure should be done for 10~15 minutes and repeated daily for seven days.

2. Electro-acupuncture is used. With the patient in a seated position, insert a 1.5cun needle into bilateral Fengchi (GB 20). Angle the needles toward the opposite ear and insert to a depth of 1.2~1.3cun. Manipulate each needle until the patient can feel the Qi sensation. Apply the electro-stimulation machine using continuous frequency waveform for 20~30 minutes. Repeat daily for ten days to complete one course of treatment.

3. Point injection is used. A 5ml syringe containing 2ml of vitamin B1, 2ml of 0.5% lidocaine and 1ml of vitamin B12 is needed. With the patient is in a seated position, locate and sterilize bilateral Fengchi (GB 20). Upon insertion, angle each needle towards the opposite ear and insert to a depth of 2.5cm. Once the depth is reached, aspirate the handle of the syringe back to be sure that no blood comes out and then inject the fluid while simultaneously withdrawing the needle. Usually one injection on each side is enough. If results are insufficient, repeat after 2-3 days.

Results

1. Method No.1: 56 cases with headaches ranging from one to more than five years in duration were treated with the acupressure method. Of these, 43 cases had functional headaches, 10 cases had hypertensive headaches, and three cases had headaches associated with dysmenorrheal: 36 cases completely resolved; 19 cases improved; and one case had no effect. All successful cases required no more than two courses of treatment.

2. Method No.2: 260 cases presented with headache from sinusitis and as a result of side-effects from medications, and were treated with one course of electro-acupuncture: 258 cases completely resolved; and two cases showed no improvement.

3. Method No.3: 50 cases presented with severe chronic headaches from head injuries, trigeminal neuralgia, or an intracranial space occupying lesion. Within four courses of point-injection treatment: 28 cases had completely resolved; 14 cases had improved slightly; and one case had no change.

Cases

1. Lai xx, male, 9-year old student: Presented with severe headache for the past six months. Clinical examination and cranial CT scan were normal. His headache improved after the first acupressure session of treatment and disappeared after the fifth session.

2. Ye xx, female, 56-year old officer: Presented with severe temporal headache of ten years duration, which increased on exposure to cold and with overwork. After three sessions of electro-acupuncture, the pain was relieved completely.

3. Tan xx, male, 41-year old teacher: Presented with persistent headache since being involved in a traffic accident six months prior. After the accident, he was hospitalized and comatose for five days until he awoke with a severe headache and nausea and vomiting. While other symptoms have improved, his headache remained. The patient was treated with the point-injection protocol every other day. After three treatments, his headache pain had vanished.

Discussion

1. The three methods above are to be used in different presentations of headache. The acupressure is best suited for mild cases, the electro-acupuncture for moderate headaches, and the point injection for severe headaches.

2. Fengchi (GB 20) is very rich in nerve supply, and is located close to important muscles of the neck, head, and primary intracranial vessels and nerves. All the methods discussed improve Qi and blood flow around Fengchi (GB 20), and thus are effective in alleviating headache.

1.2 Pain of the Supraorbital Area

This condition manifests as pain on the forehead or supraorbital bone, and can also be classified within the categories of headache or migraine. The pain is usually accompanied by local soreness, photophobia and tearing. Typically, symptoms lessen in the morning, become more intense in the afternoon and decrease in severity again in the evening.

Point

Kunlun (BL 60)

Location

Kunlun (BL 60) is located in the depression between the posterior border of the external malleolus and the Achilles tendon, at the same level as the tip of the malleolus bone.

Method

Acupuncture is used. Quickly insert a 1.5cun needle into Kunlun (BL60) on the affected side, to a depth of 1cun. Manipulate the needle using a reinforcing method in chronic cases of supraorbital pain and a reducing method in acute cases until the patient can feel a Qi sensation travel up to the knee. Then, retain the needle for 20~30 minutes and repeat manipulation every five minutes if the supraorbital pain recurs.

Results

16 cases were treated with this method and 15 cases completely resolved. Of the 15 resolved cases, 10 cases resolved after one session, three cases resolved within 2~3 sessions and two cases resolved within 3~4 sessions.

Case

Wang xx, male, 45 year old officer: Presented with supraorbital pain that was most intense in the afternoon. During treatment with the above method, the patient's pain was relieved after 15 minutes of needling. The pain did not recur after the second session.

Discussion

This type of pain usually starts in the morning. The best results can be obtained if the needle is inserted about 1/2 hour before the expected onset of pain. If the pain is chronic, using press needles on Kunlun (BL 60) can help control this situation.

1.3 Migraine

Migraines are a kind of common and severe headache, which are usually a result of genetic predisposition. Migraines often occur repeatedly, with the first onset in childhood. They are often induced by a variety of potential pathogenic factors, such as: fatigue, tension, anxiety, poor sleep or with a woman's menstrual cycle. Symptoms of migraine involve repeated attacks of intolerable burning, throbbing or boring pain of the forehead, temple and/or orbit. The pain occurs unilaterally in most cases and bilaterally in a few cases. The pain can last anywhere from a few minutes up to 1-2 days. Sometimes migraines occur several times a day and may recur every few months or few years.

Point 1

Yifeng (SJ 17)

Location

Yifeng (SJ 17) is located posterior to the ear lobe, in the depression between the mastoid process and mandibular angle.

Method

Electro-acupuncture is used. Insert a 2cun needle to a depth of 1.5cun into bilateral Yifeng (SJ 17), angling towards the point on the opposite side. Manipulate the needles using rotating and lifting techniques, focusing most on the rotating method. Most patients will feel a Qi sensation arrives in the throat and at the root of the tongue (if the needle is inserted deep enough and if the migraine pain is severe enough). Once this protocol has been applied on both points, connect the needles to an electrical stimulation machine. Use a continuous waveform for 20 to 30 minutes.

Result

150 cases were treated with this method: 76 cases completely resolved; 56 cases had marked improvement; 14 cases slightly improved and four cases had no effect. The total efficacy rate was 97.33%.

Case

Wen xx, female, 49 year-old farmer: Presented with left-sided migraine of 10-years duration, accompanied by nausea, vomiting and irritability. Her traditional Chinese medicine diagnosis was migraine due to stagnation of Qi and blood. The patient was treated with the above method, and had significant improvement after the first session. Complete relief was obtained after 10 sessions.

Discussion

Migraines are often considered a Shaoyang headache, which applies to the Sanjiao meridian. Yifeng (SJ 17) is chosen because it is on the Sanjiao meridian and is also located in the local area of the head. It has a particular function for addressing migraine by improving qi and blood flow in cervical area, and in the cranial nerves and vessels.

Point 2

Reaction point (Vesicle form)

Location

Such a phenomenon can be found in some cases of migraine, and is located on either side of the spinous processes of cervical spine. The vesicle that forms is small, and either white, light red or gray in color. It is palpable, and it does not disappear with pressure.

Method

Three-edged needling therapy is used. If the vesicle can be seen, use the needle to remove it, making a break through the skin and fiber. Repeat this for 3~5 times, then apply local anti-inflammatory medication. Cover with a plaster. Do not repeat the procedure.

If you do not see a vesicle, rub the area with your fingers, until it is palpable. If the vesicle is still undetectable, then use the extra point Dingchuan (EX-B1) for the above procedure.

Result

30 cases with migraine were treated with this method, all with good results yielded.

Case

Yin xx, female, 40 year-old worker: Presented with a one-year history of migraines accompanied by dizziness, dry mouth and insomnia. A vesicle could be found between the 3rd and 4th cervical vertebrae, 0.5cun from the spine. After the above procedure was performed, the migraine improved and disappeared after one week.

Discussion

For each disease there will be specific external signs. Vesicle therapy is specific for migraine, and the cutting with a three-edged needle regulates and improves brain function.

1.4 Trigeminal Neuralgia

Trigeminal Neuralgia is characterized by sudden attacks of spasmodic electric shock-like severe pain of the facial area supplied by the trigeminal nerve (including the ophthalmic, maxillary and mandibular divisions - but mainly along the maxillary and mandibular divisions). Attacks may recur several times per day, and most often when the patient is washing their face, brushing their teeth, eating or walking.

Point 1

Tinggong (SI 19)
(For Maxillary and Trigeminal Pain)

Location

Tinggong (SI 19) is located on the face, anterior to the tragus and posterior to the mandibular condyloid process, in the depression found when the mouth is open.

Method

Acupuncture is used. Select the point on the affected side only. Using a 30-gauge, 1.5cun needle, insert to a depth of 1cun and manipulate until the patient can feel a Qi sensation arrive on the same side as the needle. Retain the needle for up to one hour in severe cases, without manipulation. If after the first 30 minutes the pain is not relieved, you can repeat manipulation every ten minutes for the next 30 minutes.

Result

63 cases were treated with this method: 44 were completely resolved; 11 cases significantly improved; and eight cases showed slight improvement but with recurrence of the pain after one year.

Case

Li xx, male, 70 year-old worker: Presented with right facial pain of five days duration without improvement after western medical treatment. The patient showed marked improvement after three minutes of the above treatment, with the needle was further retained for one hour. After three similar sessions, the pain had completely resolved.

Discussion

This point is particularly useful for maxillary and trigeminal pain.

Point 2

Yangbi (GB 14)
(For Ophthalmic Pain)

Location

Yangbai (GB 14) is located on the forehead, directly above the pupil and 1cun above the eyebrow.

Method

Acupuncture is used. Locate the point on the affected side. Insert a 1.5cun needle horizontally and inferiorly to a depth of 1cun, inserting towards the point Yuyao (EX-HN 4)*. Manipulate the needle using a rotating technique until the arrival of a Qi sensation. Retain the needle for up to 30 minutes. The needle may also be covered with a plaster and removed the next day.

Yuyao (EX-HN 4) is in the middle of the eyebrow directly above the pupil.

1.5 Occipital Neuralgia

Occipital neuralgia refers to pain in the occipital and upper cervical area of the head and neck. It is often caused by an infectious condition, neck sprain or changes in the cervical vertebrae from C_1 to C_4. Main clinical manifestations include pain in the occipital and upper cervical areas, which is often induced by awkward movement of the neck, sneezing or cough. During an attack, the patient feels restricted movement in the neck, and pain that is mostly continuous or aggravated in paroxysmal attacks. There may also be some sharp pain even when the attack is over.

Point

Fengchi (GB 20)

Location

Fengchi (GB 20) is located on the nape of the neck, below the occipital bone, at the level of Fengfu (DU 16), in the depression between the upper ends of sternocleidomastoid and the trapezius muscles.

Method

Point injection is used. Have the patient in a seated position and prepare a 5ml syringe containing 2ml of vitamin B$_1$, 2ml of 0.5% lidocaine and 1ml of vitamin B$_{12}$. Insert needles into Fengchi (GB 20) on either side, directing them towards the opposite ear and to a depth of 2.5cm. Once the appropriate depth is reached, aspirate the syringe handle to be sure there is no blood present. Then, inject the fluid while simultaneously withdrawing the needle. Usually one injection on each side is enough. If adequate results are not achieved, the procedure may be repeated after 2-3 days.

Result

91 cases were treated with this method: 69 cases completely resolved; 20 cases markedly improved after 1-3 treatments; and two cases showed no effect after more than three treatments.

Case

Zhang xx, male, 48 years old: Presented with pain in the back of his head and neck for the past month. He had been diagnosed with occipital neuralgia and the pain presented while turning his head and when coughing. He had been given various western medications, without relief. Upon examination, Fengchi (GB 20) was notably tender. After three treatments with the above method, his symptoms had completely resolved.

Discussion

Fengchi (GB 20) is a point very rich in nerve supply, located close to important muscles of the neck, head and main intracranial vessels and nerves. All of the methods discussed improve Qi and blood flow around Fengchi (GB 20), thus alleviating headache.

1.6 Stiff Neck

A "stiff neck" occurs when the neck muscles become strained as a result of exposure to cold, sleeping on high pillows, or excessive and prolonged tilting to one side. Usually, a stiff neck manifests with pain and limited movement of the neck.

Two points can be used in the treatment of stiff neck: Xuanzhong (GB 39) and Houxi (SI 3).

Point 1

Xuanzhong (GB 39)

Location

Xuanzhong (GB 39) is located on the lateral side of the leg, 3cun above the tip of external malleolus, on the anterior border of the fibula.

Method

Acupuncture is used. With the patient in a seated position, expose the points bilaterally. Insert a 1.5~2cun needle at each point to a depth of 1.2~1.8cun, depending on the size of the patient. Stimulate the point strongly, until the patient can feel a Qi sensation travelling up to the knee. Simultaneously, the patient should stretch and rotate their neck to loosen the muscles. Retain the needles for 15~20 minutes, repeating manipulation every five minutes.

Result

74 cases were treated with this method: 43 cases completely resolved (41 resolved after one treatment, and two cases after two treatments); three cases significantly improved after two treatments; and one case did not improve.

Case

Zhao xx, male, 27 years old: Presented with right-sided neck pain as a result of a poor sleeping position. The pain was accompanied by tenderness and stiffness of the neck muscles and an inability to tilt the neck to the right side. Massage therapy offered no relief. The diagnosis was stiff neck. Within 20 minutes of the above acupuncture treatment, the pain had significantly improved.

Discussion

Xuanzhong (GB 39) belongs to the gallbladder meridian, which flows through the neck. Inserting the needle at Xuanzhong (GB 39) improves Qi and blood along the gallbladder meridian, thus alleviating neck pain and stiffness.

Point 2

Houxi (SI 3)

Location

Houxi (SI 3) is located at the junction of the red and white skin along the ulnar border of the hand, at the ulnar end of the distal palmar crease, proximal to the 5th metacarpophalangeal joint when a hollow fist is made.

Method

Acupuncture is used. With the patient in the sitting position, select the points on both sides. Insert a 1.5cun needle towards Hegu (LI 4), at a depth exceeding 1cun. Rotate the needle using a reducing method for 1~3 minutes, until the patient feels no more neck pain. Then, remove the needle. If the pain was not relieved, retain the needles for 20~30 minutes and repeat manipulation every five minutes.

Result

54 cases were treated with this method: 33 cases completely resolved; 19 cases improved; and two cases showed no effect. Most of the improved cases needed 1~2 sessions of treatment.

Case

Xao xx, male, 37 years old: Presented with neck stiffness, which was worse in the morning. The pain radiated to the right side of the shoulder, and worsened when tilting the neck to the left side. The diagnosis was stiff neck. After three minutes of needle manipulation using the above method, the pain had relieved.

1.7 Cervical Spondylopathy

Cervical spondylopathy occurs when a hyper-osteogenesis (bone-spur) of the cervical vertebra stimulates or oppresses the cervical nerve root, spinal cord, vertebral artery or sympathetic nerve. The condition causes pain, limited movement or other symptoms. The main clinical manifestations are soreness, distension or pain of the neck, shoulder or arm; numbness of the fingers; and others. It is a condition usually seen in those over the age of forty.

Point

Changshanxia (Experiential Point)

Location

Changshanxia (experiential point) is located 2cun below the point Chengshan (BL 57), and slightly interior, according to the site of tenderness upon palpation. Chengshan (BL 57) is located on the posterior midline of the leg, between Weizhong (BL 40) and Kunlun (BL 60), in a depression formed below the gastrocnemius muscle belly when the leg is stretched or the heel is lifted (See Fig. 1-1).

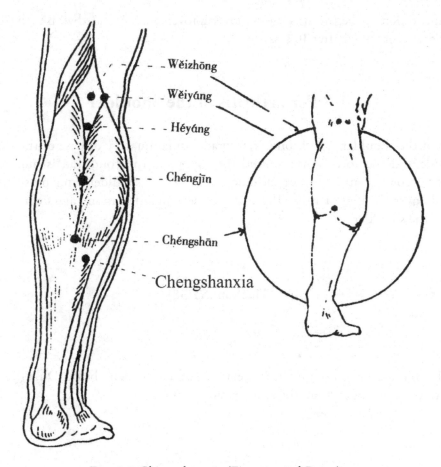

Fig. 1-1 Changshanxia (Experiential Point)

Method

Acupuncture, cupping and massage are used. With the patient in a prone position, locate the point on both sides, according to local tenderness. Insert a 1.5 cun perpendicularly and manipulate it until the patient feels a local Qi sensation. Then, cover the needle with a cup. After 15 minutes, remove the needle and the cup and start massaging, first using both hands to relax all of the leg muscles. Continue massaging with the thumb around the local area, and running up the leg. Repeat upward rubbing for 20-30 minutes, until the patient feels muscle distention in the area, the neck feels hot to the touch and with slight perspiration. The patient should simultaneously move their neck throughout the entire treatment.

Result

10 or more treatments are required for complete resolution.

Case

Luo xx, male, 45 years old: Presented with neck pain and numbness in both hands. Upon inserting the needles, the patient noticed a heat sensation from the low back up to the neck and along the shoulder and hand. In addition, he began to sweat. Steady improvement continued with each treatment, and complete relief was obtained after 10 sessions.

1.8 Periarthritis of the Shoulder

Periarthritis of the shoulder is a chronic, retrograde, inflammatory disease of the shoulder joint, should capsule and the soft tissues around the shoulder. The condition is most often caused by exposure to cold, trauma and/or chronic strain of the shoulder, and most often presents in individuals over the age of fifty. The main clinical manifestations are soreness and limited movement of the shoulder.

Point

Tiaokou (ST 38)

Location

Tiaohou (ST 38) is located on the anterior-lateral side of the leg, 8cun below Dubi (ST 35), and one finger-breadth (middle finger) from the anterior crest of tibia.

Methods

1. Acupuncture is used. With the patient in a seated position, insert a 1.5-2.5cun needle into Tiaohou (ST 38) on the affected side. Stimulate the point strongly by lifting and rotating for about 3 minutes until the patient can feel a Qi sensation. Retain the needles for 20 minutes, continuing manipulation for 2-3 rounds. Repeat sessions every 1-2 days until the patient can easily move the shoulder without pain.

2. Piercing needling therapy is used. With the patient in a seated position, expose Tiaokuo (ST 38) on the affected side. Use a needle with a gauge 26 or 28 (thick needle), and 3-4cun long. Insert the needle at Tiaokuo (ST 38) directed forwards Chengshan (BL 57) to a depth of 2.5-3.5 cun. Manipulate the needle by rotating it counter-clockwise until the patient feels a Qi sensation moving up the arm and shoulder. Simultaneously, have the patient moves their shoulder joint in any direction. Once a strong sensation is obtained, retain the needles for 15 minutes, manipulating 2-3 more times. Repeat the treatment every 1-2 days.

3. Point injection is used. Prepare a 5ml syringe containing 1ml of vitamin B12, 2 ml of 0.5% lidocaine and 1ml of vitamin B1. Bilaterally locate the point Tiaokuo (ST 38) and inject 2 ml of the mixture at a depth of 2.0 cm on either side (even if shoulder pain is unilateral). Repeat this procedure 1-2 times per week. Simultaneously during treatment, flash cupping may be applied at Ashi (tender) points on the shoulder.

Results

1. 34 cases were treated with the first method: 13 cases completely resolved; 16 cases markedly improved; three cases slightly improved; and two cases showed no change.

2. 45 cases were treated with the second method: 38 cases completely resolved; three cases slightly improved; and four cases had no effect.

3. 53 cases were treated with the third method: all yielded good results within 1-3 weeks of treatment.

Cases

1. Wang xx, male, 52 year-old officer: Presented with pain and limited mobility of the right shoulder. Many Western medications and therapies had been tried, without relief. The traditional Chinese medicine diagnosis was periarthritis of the shoulder due to wind and damp. After four acupuncture treatments with the above protocol, his symptoms had resolved completely.

2. Gao xx, female, 52 years old: Presented with right shoulder pain and limited movement for the past two months. After one session of piercing needle therapy, she had marked improvement in her symptoms. After four sessions, her pain had alleviated completely.

3. Huang xx, female, 54 years old: Presented with chronic right shoulder pain for the past 10 years, which was diagnosed as periarthritis of the shoulder. She had tried many Western medications without any effect. After six treatments of point injection therapy, her symptoms had greatly improved.

Discussion

1. The point Tiaokuo (ST 38) belongs to stomach meridian of Foot Yangming. Among the twelve regular meridians, the Yangming meridians are the richest in Qi and blood. Tiaokuo (ST 38) can improve blood and Qi flow efficiently in the stomach meridian all the way up to the shoulder. Shoulder movement also relieves stagnation of blood and encourages the flow of Qi, thus relieving pain and limited range of movement.

2. The needle may be inserted at Tiaokuo (ST 38) or at a tender point around it - but no more than 1cun away from the actual point. Just lateral to the point is typically the most painful and tender point. Both sides should be checked for which is most tender.

3. The point Tiaokuo (ST 38) is experientially known to alleviate referred tenderness of the shoulder joint.

4. Between acupuncture sessions, the patient should exercise the shoulder at home for 30 minutes, 2-3 times daily.

1.9 Brachialgia

Brachialgia refers to specific and severe pain of the shoulder joint alone (not in the arm and elbow), followed by motor weakness. Sensory loss is usually minimal and it is due to either a brachial plexus injury by traction, penetrating wounds or compression. The upper part of the brachial plexus is commonly more affected than the lower part.

Point

Futu (LI 18)

Location

Futu (LI 18) is located on the lateral side of the neck, beside the laryngeal protuberance and between the anterior and posterior borders of the sternocleidonastiod muscle.

Method

Acupuncture is used. Use the point on the affected side. Insert a 1cun needle into the point, directed towards the cervical spine and to a depth no more than 0.5 cun (to avoid injury of the carotid artery). Once the patient can feel a Qi sensation move down their arm, remove the needle - do not retain it. Repeat this procedure daily for up to 10 days.

Result

123 cases were treated with this method: 92 cases completely resolved; 26 cases slightly improved; and five cases did not improve at all.

Case

Shu xx, male, 59 year-old farmer: Presented with left shoulder pain with limited arm movement, which developed upon exposure to rainy weather. The diagnosis was brachialgia. After five treatments with the above method, the pain markedly improved. By the end of the 7th treatment, the arm was able to move freely.

Discussion

The point Futu (LI 18) belongs to the hand Yangming meridian, which flows through the arms and around the shoulder. Stimulation of this point can improve Qi and blood flow in shoulder and arm.

1.10 Tennis Elbow

Tennis elbow, also called lateral humeral epicondylitis, manifests itself as pain at the origin of the common tendon of the forearm extensors, on the lateral side of the elbow joint. Tennis elbow is caused by laceration, bleeding, adhesion or aseptic inflammatory changes of the tendon attached to the main extensor muscle of the elbow joint from chronic strain. It manifests as pain in the lateral side of the elbow, and may radiate to the shoulder and/or wrist. The affected arm feels sore and weak, often changing in severity.

Point

Ashi point

Location

This Ashi point is located in the center of the lateral epicondyle of the humerus.

Methods

1. Moxibustion with ginger is used. Have the patients seated with their arms resting on a table and the elbows flexed. Palpate for Ashi points around the elbow. Take the fresh ginger and rub it around the skin of the Ashi point until the local area of skin becomes little red. Apply a small piece of Musk (a kind of Chinese pharmaceutical, use a size similar to a piece of rice) on the Ashi point. Slice a piece of ginger 0.3cun thick by 3-4cun in diameter, and place it over the Musk on the Ashi point. Secure the ginger to the skin using surgical tape, leaving the center of the ginger slice uncovered. Be sure that the tape is tightly sealed around the skin and ginger so that no air can escape through plaster edges. Ignite a moxa stick and apply it as near as 3cun from ginger until the patient can feel the local area becoming comfortably warm (but not too hot). One session should last for 10 minutes. Keep the plaster, ginger and Musk at the site until the next session, remove the plaster and ginger and repeat the entire procedure daily for 10 days.

2. Intradermal needling is used. Insert an intradermal needle with a 0.5cun handle horizontally into the Ashi point - between the skin and muscle and in the direction of the muscle fibers. Secure the needle with surgical tape, and ask the patient to move the elbow until the patient feels comfortable and without pain. Retain the needle for 3-5 days, then remove.

3. Dermal needle (plum-blossom needle or Seven-star needle) is used. Tap the Ashi point at the elbow with such a device until a little blood comes out. Then, apply moxa until the skin becomes red in color (as in method 1). Repeat every other day, until the patient feels improvement.

Results

1. *Method 1 - Moxibustion with Ginger.* 100 cases were treated: 70 cases completely resolved; 17 cases had marked improvement; 15 cases slightly improved; and three cases had no effect.

2. *Method 2 - Intradermal Needle.* 25 cases were treated: 16 cases completely resolved (12 resolved within one session, and four within two sessions); and nine cases slightly improved.

3. *Method 3 - Dermal Needling.* 15 cases were treated: all improved within 2~3 sessions.

Cases

1. Zhang xx, male, 38 year-old worker: Presented with right elbow pain accompanied by limited movement of the elbow joint. The pain increased with movement and when exposed to cold. After three courses of moxibustion with ginger treatment, the pain had markedly improved.

2. Feng xx, male, 58 years old: Presented with right elbow pain of one-month duration, which increased upon moving the elbow, after three days of retained intradermal needle therapy, he showed marked improvement.

3. Peng xx, male, 23 years old: Presented with right elbow pain of five days duration, which worsened with movement. After applying the third method for two sessions, the condition had improved significantly.

Discussion

Tennis Elbow results from repetitive strain of the elbow joint or exposure to cold, both resulting a deficiency of Qi and stagnation of blood. All of the methods explained above are used to promote the flow of Qi and alleviate stagnation of blood.

1.11 Wrist and Ankle Sprain

A wrist or ankle sprain occurs from injury and the main clinical manifestations include local pain, swelling and limitation of movement in the affected joint.

Point

Relative point

Location

To locate the relative point, first find a tender or Ashi point on the injured ankle or wrist. Then, find the corresponding area on the opposite ankle or wrist from the injury - which will be the relative point. If the ankle is injured, the relative point corresponds to the tender point on the ankle transposed onto the wrist. On the contrary, if wrist is injured, select the relative point on the ankle.

Method

Acupuncture is used. Select the relative points on the affected side of the body. Insert a 1 cun needle at the relative point, angled obliquely and proximally upward to a depth of 0.5~0.8 cun. Manipulate the needle with a reducing method - using lifting, thrusting and rotating techniques until the patient can feel a Qi sensation. The patient should simultaneously move the injured joint during this procedure. The needle should be retained for 20~30 minutes, If the pain recurs, repeat manipulation very five minutes. For joint swelling, apply local anti inflammatory pharmaceuticals and cover with plaster.

Result

40 cases (15 with wrist and 25 with ankle injury) were treated with this method. All of the cases had pain with swelling and limited joint movement. All of the cases improved after one treatment.

Case

Bai xx, male, 40 year-old, officer: Presented with right ankle sprain, which occurred while walking downstairs. The ankle was swollen, painful, and had limited movement. Upon X-ray, the joint appeared normal and he was diagnosed with an ankle sprain. While manipulating the relative point on the right wrist for 15 minutes, the pain had much improved. After three sessions, the discomfort had completely resolved.

Discussion

Relative points are located far away from the site of injury, which is useful since the nature of the internal trauma is unknown. Any needle insertion at local area may exacerbate a hidden structural injury. Utilizing the wrists and ankles for this purpose falls under the category of micro-acupuncture therapy, as they relate to each other through meridians and collaterals. It is therefore that pain in one joint can be treated by manipulation of the relative point on the other joint.

1.12 Shoulder and Back Pain

Shoulder and back pain can originate from arthritis or any number of local inflammations of the tendons and muscles. The main manifestations are limitation of movement and pain and tenderness over the affected area.

Point

Shangshandian (Experiential Point)

Location

Shangshandian (experiential point) is located by drawing a line 3cun posterior from the thyroid cartilage, then continuing perpendicularly downward for 1cun. The point is located within the sternocleidomastiod muscle (See Fig. 1-2).

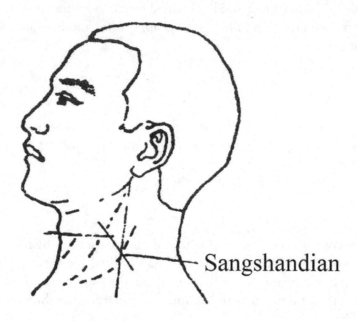

Fig. 1-2 Shangshandian (Experiential Point)

Method

Acupuncture is used. Select the point on the affected side. Insert a 28 guage-1.5cun needle to a maximum depth of 0.5cun. Manipulate the needle by lifting and thrusting quickly, yet with small amplitude, until the patient can feel a Qi sensation. The best effect is obtained when the patient feels the Qi sensation travel down to their fingers. Once a Qi sensation is felt remove the needle. Do not retain the needle.

Result

246 cases were treated with this method: 133 cases completely resolved; 122 cases had some improvement; and nine cases did not respond.

Case

Zhao xx, female, 59 years old: Presented with hemiplegia accompanied by shoulder and back pain for the past six months. After her first treatment with the above method, her pain had reduced. After ten treatments her arm began to regain power.

1.13. Intercostal Neuralgia

Intercostal neuralgia is characterized by a prickling or lacerating pain along the region of distribution of the intercostal nerve. Other manifestations include frequent pain within one or more intercostal spaces, sometimes with a belt like distribution. The pain is intensified by coughing or deep breathing, and is characterized by a sharp pricking or electric shock-like sensation.

Point

Qiuxu (GB 40)

Location

Qiuxu (GB 40) is located anterior and inferior to the external malleolus, in the depression lateral to the tendon of the long extensor muscle of toes.

Method

Acupuncture is used. Select the point Qiuxu (GB 40) on the contra lateral side. Insert a 1.5cun needle to a depth of 1.0cun and rotate the needle until the patient can feel a local Qi sensation. The needle should then be retained for 30 minutes, manipulating every 10 minutes. Repeat the treatment every day.

Result

44 cases were treated with this method: 33 cases completely resolved; eight cases improved; and three cases did not show any improvement. Most of the improved cases showed optimal effect after six sessions.

Case

Yang xx, male, 17 year-old student: Presented with burning right-sided chest pain accompanied with tenderness along the mid-clavicular line from the 4th to the 6th rib. The patient had not responded to any other medical treatment. The traditional Chinese medicine diagnosis was intercostal neuralgia due to stagnation of blood. His symptoms began to improve after the first acupuncture session, and were completely resolved after eight sessions.

Discussion

The intercostal space belongs to the Shaoyang meridians. Qiuxu (GB 40) is the primary Yuan source point on the gall bladder meridian of Foot Shaoyang. Manipulation of Qiuxu (GB 40) improves Qi and blood flow in this region.

1.14 Lumbar Transverse Process Syndrome

Lumbar transverse process syndrome refers to local muscle injury caused by aseptic swelling, hyperemia and exudation, which leads to proliferation of the periosteum and fibrous tissue. Clinical manifestations include pain in the lower back, which radiates to the ipsilateral leg, and is aggravated by movement.

Point

Ashi Point

Location

The Ashi point is located in the center of the most painful area in the lumbar region.

Method

Acupuncture and cupping therapy are used. Have the patient lie in a prone position with a small pillow beneath the abdomen. Select the Ashi points on the affected side. Insert a 3cun needle to a depth of 2cun and manipulate using a reducing method. Once the patient can feel a Qi sensation, cover the needle with the vacuum-sealed cup and retain for 20 minutes. Repeat every-other-day, and one treatment course equals six sessions.

Result

85 cases were treated with this method: 61 cases completely resolved; 22 cases improved; and two cases did not show improvement.

Case

Zhou xx, male, 27 year-old soldier: Presented with low back pain that began while carrying a gun on his shoulder. An X-ray film showed he had an injury at the transverse process on his L3 vertebrae. The diagnosis was third lumbar vertebra transverse process syndrome. The patient was treated with the above method with the Ashi point inserted 1.5cun just lateral to the spine. After three sessions, he showed complete improvement.

Discussion

The transverse process of L3 is relatively long, protruding outwards, and not sufficiently covered by muscles to protect it - and is therefore easily injured. Acupuncture and cupping improve Qi and blood flow in the local area, thus relieving the pain.

1.15 Acute Lumbar Muscle Sprain

Acute lumbar pain is a common symptom caused by traumatic sprain of the lumbar region, muscular strain in the lumbar region, or rheumatic myotitis of the lumbar muscles. This disease is mostly due to improper posture, falling, wrestling, sprains or contusions that in turn damage the lumbar muscles, fascias, and ligaments. The main clinical manifestations are persistent back pain with stiffness of the lumbar spine, local tenderness and limited movement of the lumbar spine.

One of two points may be used, Yinjiao (DU 28) or Yaotong (EX-UE 7), an extra point.

Point 1

Yinjiao (DU 28)

Location

Yinjiao (DU 28) is located on the inside of the upper lip, at the junction of the labial frenulum and the upper gum.

Method

Three-edged needle therapy is used. In most cases of acute lumbar pain, a small vesicle can be detected on the labial frenulum about 12 hours after the onset of pain. The vesicle will be white or a deep-red color. Have the patient in a seated position with the neck hyper-extended back. Lift the upper lip and insert the three-edged needle into the center of the vesicle, then quickly remove it. If excess blood comes out, apply a little white sugar topically. Once the procedure is done accurately, there should be no need to repeat.

Result

174 cases were treated with this method: 148 cases completely resolved; 25 cases slightly improved; and one case did not improve. In most cases, the procedure was done only once.

Case

Chui xx, male, 50 year-old worker: Presented with acute lumbar pain after lifting heavy objects two days prior. A small vesicle was removed from under his lip and the pain decreased significantly. By the next day, he had no more pain.

Discussion

1. Yinjiao (DU 28) is interconnected with the Ren meridian and belongs to the Du Meridian. The Du meridian controls all of the Yang meridians; while the Ren meridian controls all of the Yin meridians. As the Du meridian follows the midline of the back, it supplies the back

with Qi and blood. Hence, removing the vesicle relieves stagnation of Qi and blood in the back, thus alleviating lumbar pain.

2.   If you do not own a three-edged needle or you cannot use it properly, use a syringe (hypodermic) needle to remove the vesicle.

Point 2

Yaotongdian (EX-UE 7)

Location

Yaotongdian (EX-UE 7) refers to two points on the dorsum of each hand, between the 1st and 2nd and also between the 3rd and 4th metacarpal bones, and at the midpoint between the dorsal crease of the wrist and metacarpophalangeal joints (See Fig. 1-3).

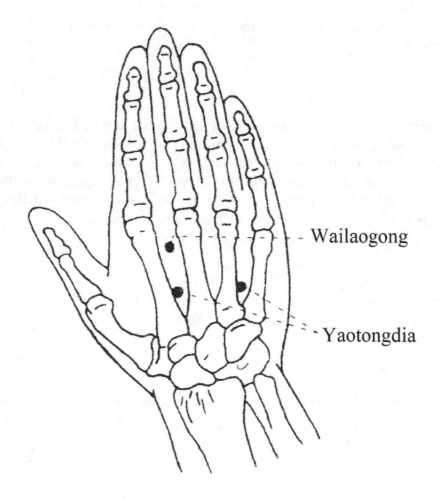

Fig. 1-3 Yaotongdian (EX-UE 7)

22

Method

Acupuncture is used. Manual stimulation of Yaotongdian (EX- UE 7) is used in cases of acute lumbar pain when no vesicle inside the upper lip can be found. Use the points on the affected side. Insert a 26 gauge-1cun needle to a depth of 0.3~0.4cun and stimulate them strongly until the patient can feel a Qi sensation in their back. Meanwhile, ask the patient to simultaneously move their back muscles by bending and rotating the waist.

Result

120 cases were treated with this method: 58 cases completely resolved; 43 cases significantly improved; and 19 cases slightly improved.

Case

Shen xx, male, 17 year-old student: Presented in the clinic after a low back injury while playing basketball at school. The initial symptoms included pain and stiffness of the lower back and the local skin was hot to the touch. Upon viewing the X-ray, it was apparent that all bones were intact and the problem was an acute muscular sprain in his low back. The pain had decreased after his first acupuncture treatment, and completely relieved after the second visit.

1.16 Chronic Lumbar Muscle Strain

Chronic lumbar muscle strain happens when the lumbar muscles are intensely strained in a continuous or repeated manner over a short period of time, which exceeds the person's physiological endurance and therefore results in chronic aseptic inflammation of the lumbar muscle fibers. The occurrence of such pathology is closely related to dampness in traditional Chinese medicine. For example, if someone lives in a damp room or basement, or lies down on damp ground, they may be more prone to this condition. It manifests itself as long-term pain of the lumbar, affecting either one or both sides. The pain is typically aggravated when the patient is tired, and relieved upon gentle activity.

Point

Pigen (EX-B4)

Location

Pigen (EX-B4), is an extra point located on the low back, below the spinous process of the 1st lumbar vertebra and 3.5 cun lateral to the posterior midline (See Fig. 1-4).

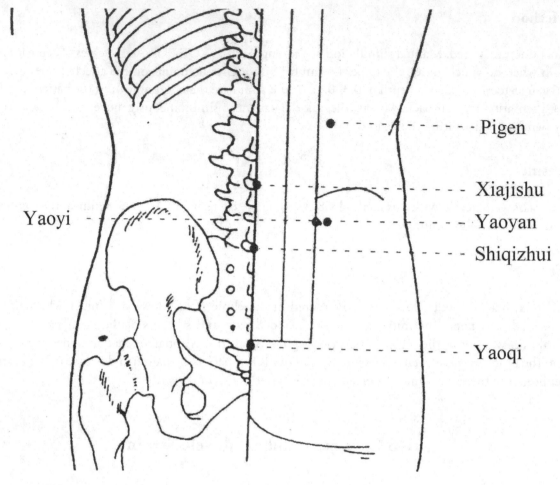

Fig. 1-4 Pigen (EX-B4)

Method

Acupuncture, moxibustion and cupping are used. Locate the point on both sides, with the patient lying down in a prone position. Obliquely insert a 3cun needle (at an angle of 45°) to a depth of 2~2.5cun - until the patient can feel a Qi sensation traveling down toward their knee. Apply pole moxa around the needle until the local area is red with a little sweating and retain the needle for 20 minutes. Then, apply a cup over the needle and leave for another 10 minutes. Repeat daily, one treatment course is 8 sessions.

Result

100 cases were treated with this method: 82 cases completely resolved; 11 cases improved; and seven cases did not show any effect. All patients were treated for 1~10 sessions, with the average being 5 sessions.

Case

Zhou xx, male, 56 years old: Presented with chronic, recurrent low back pain with limited range of movement and local stiffness in the mornings. His X-ray showed a normal spine. The traditional Chinese medicine diagnosis was chronic lumbar muscle strain due to stagnation of blood. He was treated with the above method and his pain had markedly improved after 10 treatments

Discussion

Chronic lumbar muscle strain is mainly due to trauma, or any of the external pathogenic factors that can injure the kidneys: wind, cold or damp. The Kidney meridian is closely related to the extra meridians. Pigen (EX-B4) is located along the pathway of an extra meridian and stimulation of the point even by acupressure can greatly alleviate pain.

1.17 Sciatica

Sciatica is a kind of radiating and continuous pain along the sciatic nerve distribution, which includes the hip region, the posterior lateral aspect of the thigh and leg, and the lateral aspect of the foot. Depending on individual etiology, sciatica can be divided into primary and secondary types. Primary sciatica can be the result of various infections (such as influenza, rheumatism, malaria, syphilis, brucellosis, tuberculosis), from intoxication (for instance, by an alcohol), because of metabolic concerns (gout, diabetes, vitamin deficiency), as well as injuries. Secondary sciatica is also called sciatic neuritis or symptomatic sciatica. This type is caused mainly by pathological stimulation, either by pressure or injury to the adjacent nerves near to the sciatic nerve (such as vertebral or disc problems). Secondary sciatica is a more common presentation than primary sciatica.

Point

Shuangyang (Experiential Point)

Location

Shuangyang (experiential point) is located by drawing a straight line between Huantiao (GB 30) and Fengshi (GB 31). From the midpoint of that line, go posterior and perpendicular for 1cun. The two Shuangyang points are located 1cun above and 1cun below the point found in the previous instruction. The points lie between the gall bladder and urinary bladder meridians. *{N.B: Huantiao (GB 30) is located at the junction of the lateral 1/3 and medial 2/3 of the distance between the great trochanter and the hiatus of the sacrum. Locate this point while the patient is in the lateral position with the hip flexed. Fengshi (GB 31) is located on the midline of the lateral aspect of the thigh, 7 cun above the transverse popliteal crease}* (See Fig. 1-5).

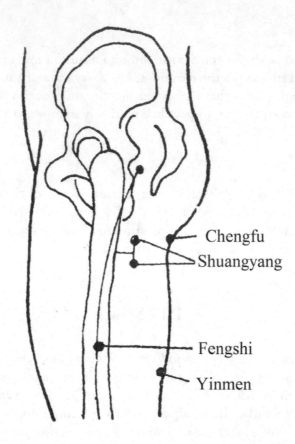

Fig. 1-5 Shuangyang (Experiential Point)

Method

Acupuncture, moxibustion and cupping are used. Select the Shuangyang points on the affected side and an insert 3cun needle into each point, directing them towards each other and each to depth of 2.5cun. Strongly manipulate the needles by lifting and rotating until the patient can feel a Qi sensation going down to their foot. Then, apply pole moxa until the local area becomes red. Retain the needles for 20 more minutes. Then, apply flash cupping over the area and leave the cups over the points for 10 minutes. Repeat daily.

Result

44 cases were treated with this method: 27 cases completely resolved; 11 cases markedly improved; and two cases did not show improvement.

Case

Wang xx, female, 45 year old farmer: Presented with chronic low back and leg pain, accompanied by limited movement and coldness of the leg. The traditional Chinese medicine diagnosis was sciatica due to cold and damp. After 10 sessions of the above treatment protocol, her symptoms had completely improved.

Discussion

Sciatica is mainly due to wind, cold and damp, so moxa and cupping are quite effective methods. The Shangyang points relate to the roots of the sciatic nerve, and the main muscles and vessels around it. Stimulating this point can improve sciatic pain, low back pain and leg pain - sciatica is merely only one of this point's treatable conditions.

1.18 Pain in Lower Back and Leg

Pain in lower back and leg is a common clinical symptom. It is often caused by sciatica, lumbar sprain, hyperplasia of the lumbar vertebrae or prolapse of a lumbar intervertebral disc. Main clinical manifestations include pain radiating from the lumbar region to the foot and limited range of motion that improves with movement.

Point

Xiashandian (Experiential Point)

Location

Xiashandian point is an experiential point found by drawing a straight line between Zhibian (BL 54) and Huantiao (GB 30). This line forms the "base" of an equilateral triangle. Xiashandian is at the apex of this triangle, which is directed posterior in relation to the base (See Fig. 1-6).

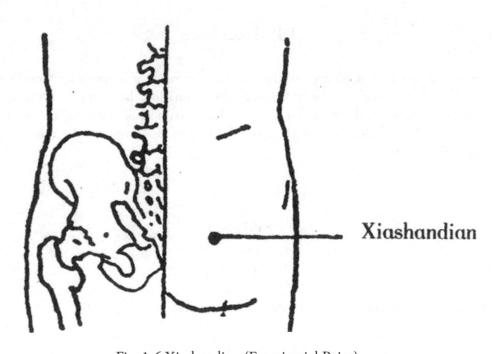

Fig. 1-6 Xiashandian (Experiential Point)

Method

Acupuncture is used. Have the patient lie lateral-recumbent on the side contra-lateral to the pain. Locate the point on the affected side. Insert a 3~4cun needle to a depth of 2.5~3.5cun. Manipulate the needle by quickly lifting and thrusting, until the patient can feel a Qi sensation going down to their foot. Repeat daily.

Result

259 cases were treated with this method, and all cases completely resolved: 184 cases required one session; 61 cases required two sessions; and 14 cases required three sessions.

Case

Wang xx, male, 30 year-old worker: Presented with lower back and leg pain, which developed after falling down while lifting heavy object. The pain and tenderness was located at the 4th and 5th sacral vertebrae. The lumbosacral spine appeared normal upon X-ray and he was diagnosed with lumbar sprain. After one treatment by the above method, all of his discomfort was relieved.

Discussion

Xiashandian (experiential point) is also effective for pain and numbness of the thigh. If the patient does not feel the Qi sensation during the procedure, it will be of no value. It is also recommended that individuals with the above presentation avoid cold and exercise during treatment.

1.19 Heel Pain

Heel pain is due to either tendonitis of the Achilles tendon or a pathological condition of the calcaneum (heel bone) such as: chronic sprain, inflammation, bone spur, or prolapse of the calcaneum. Symptoms usually manifest as general foot pain upon walking and with palpable tenderness along the affected side of the foot, the sole of the foot and the area distal to the calcaneum (Ashi points).

Point

Ashi point

Location

This Ashi point is located on the most-tender spot of the heel.

Methods

1. Massage therapy is used. With the patient lying supine and the leg muscles relaxed, massage the tender area for 10 minutes. Proper technique involves rubbing and rolling the fingers. Repeat daily for 10 sessions.

2. Moxibustion therapy is used. Rub the Ashi point with fresh ginger, then apply a new piece of fresh ginger on the affected area. Ignite a moxa cone and place it directly over the ginger. Use 3-5 cones each treatment. One course equals 10 treatment sessions.

Result

115 cases were treated with moxa and massage: 102 cases completely resolved; eight cases improved; and five cases did not show any effect.

Case

Qian xx, male, 54 years old: Presented with right heel pain, which worsened on exposure to cold weather and was accompanied by a cold sensation and numbness of the right foot. The X-ray film revealed a calcaneum (heel) spur and the official diagnosis was prolapse of the calcaneum. He was treated with both of the above methods and his symptoms dramatically improved after two treatments.

1.20 Knee pain

Aside from arthritis, sudden movements such as falls or unexpected pressure can cause lesions on soft tissues (muscles, tendons or ligaments), leading to pain of the knee. Clinical manifestations include pain, tenderness, swelling and limited of movement of the knee joint.

Point

Xiyan (EX-LE 5)

Location

Xiyan (EX-LE 5) is a pair of extra points located in the depressions on either side of the patellar ligament, when the knee is flexed. The medial and lateral points are named "Neixiyan" and "Waixiyan" respectively (See Fig 1-7).

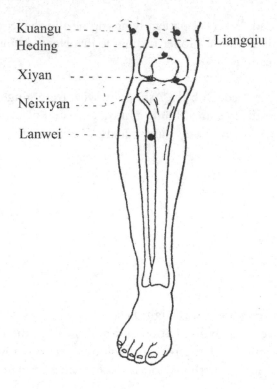

Fig 1-7 Xiyan (EX-LE 5)

Method

Electric-acupuncture is used. Have the patient lie down in a supine position with a pillow beneath the knee to keep it flexed at 120°. Insert needles into the medial and lateral Xiyan (EX-LE 5) points to a depth of 1.0~1.5cun. Angle the needles towards the center of the knee until the patient can feel a Qi sensation in the area. Then, connect the needles to an electric stimulation machine set at continuous wave frequency - set at the patient's maximum tolerance level. Leave for 30 minutes and repeat the procedure everyday or every other day.

Result

146 cases were treated with this method: 120 cases completely resolved; 16 cases markedly improved; 11 cases slightly improved; and six cases had no improvement. The total success rate was 95.89%, and most of the patients improved after the first treatment.

Case

Hu xx, male, 54 year-old farmer: Presented with chronic recurrent knee pain, which worsened upon exposure to cold and was accompanied by redness of the skin and limited knee movement. The patient was diagnosed with arthritis of the knee. He was treated by the above method and after the first treatment he felt much better. After eight sessions, the pain had disappeared altogether.

Discussion

1. The exterior Xiyan (EX-LE 5) point pertains to the stomach meridian, which is the richest in Qi and blood among the 12 regular meridians. Applying the electric machine to these points ensures that the flow of Qi and blood within the knee is optimally maintained, thus having a stronger effect on alleviating symptoms.

2. Having the knee flexed at 120° during the procedure is important to avoid painful insertion of the needle and to allow the needle to smoothly enter deep into the center of the joint.

1.21 General pain

General pain refers to pain at any part of the body, or all over the body. The pain may be due to a diagnosed or developing disease, such as: chronic pain, chronic fatigue or fibrolyalgia. If the pain is continuous, the patient will often also feel tired, restless and/or have insomnia.

Point

Ear Apex (MA-H 6)

Location

Ear apex (MA-H 6) is an auricular point located at the top of the helix, opposite to the posterior border of superior Antihelix Crus (See page 203 Auricular points picture).

Method

Acupuncture is used. Locate the point on both sides. Insert a 1cun needle to a depth of 0.3~0.5cun, directing it downward and posterior. Rotate the needle gently until the patient can feel a burning sensation in the local area of the ear. Retain the needle for 20~30 minutes, and repeat manipulation every 10 minutes. In severe cases, or if the pain continues to reoccur, the needles may be retained for 2~3 days (then changed). One course of treatment consists of 6~8 sessions.

Result

87 cases with different types of pain were treated with this method: 48 cases completely resolved; 34 cases improved; and 25 cases did not respond. The total improvement rate was 94.6%.

Discussion

This method is suitable for headache, sciatica, shoulder and arm pain, low back pain (including lumbago), rheumatic and rheumatoid arthritis, rheumatic myositis, intercostal neuralgia, visceral pain, post operative pain and pain associated with some cancers. The pain is usually relieved within five minutes and this method is known to be four times more potent than any other analgesic.

1.22 Angina Pectoris

Angina pectoris refers to colic pain in the heart, caused by chronic coronary insufficiency or acute myocardial ischemia. In general, angina pectoris is associated with coronary heart disease. The main clinical manifestations include chest pain radiating to the left back and shoulder or to the medial side of the left arm. The sudden onset of symptoms is often induced by extreme fatigue, excessive eating, and exposure to extreme cold or excitement. The symptoms usually last for 3-6 minutes and can often be alleviated by rest or medication. It is important to note that the treatment below is meant to significantly reduce the symptoms while the patient is en route to emergency medical care for proper evaluation of the cause of the angina.

Point

Zhiyang (DU 9)

Location

Zhiyang (DU 9) is located on the back, and on the posterior midline, in the depression below the spinous process of the 7th thoracic vertebra.

Methods

1. Acupressure is used. Position the patient sitting down and leaning forwards onto a table or chair. When the chest pain occurs, press perpendicularly onto the point Zhiyang (DU 9) with the edge of a small coin until the chest pain decreases or vanishes.

2. Intradermal needle therapy is used. Insert a 0.5-1.0cun intradermal needle into the point Zhiyang (DU 9) and cover it with plaster. If the pain recurs, instruct the patient to have someone press with their finger tip on the point (DU 9). Change the needle every 3-4 days. One course of treatment is 6-8 sessions. *(NB: The pain relief after pressure or retained needle should last up to 40 minutes).*

Results

1. 40 cases were treated with method one: 39 cases improved and one case had no improvement.

2. 26 cases were treated with the second method: 23 cases markedly improved; two cases had slight improvement; and one case remained the same.

Discussion

1. Angina pectoris is due to deficiency or stagnation of Yang Qi and blood. The Du meridian controls all the Yang meridians in the body. The stimulation of the point Zhiyang (DU 9) can improve Qi and blood flow within all the other Yang meridians.

2. According to the theory of relationship to organ location, the point Zhiyang (DU 9) is directly behind the heart, and is thus, specific for coronary pain.

3. Manipulating the point Zhiyang (DU 9) by pressing with a coin edge, can also be used diagnostically for coronary pain. If the pain disappears upon pressure, then it is due to coronary heart disease (the reverse is also true).

4. Pressing with a coin is a simple procedure that can be done at home, especially, if pain recurs frequently. Additionally, any object with a pointed tip or edge (such as a cup) can be placed on a bed with the patient lying down so that the edge sits just beneath the point Zhiyang (DU 9).

1.23 Cholecystalgia

Cholecystalgia refers to acute gallbladder pain. It is usually caused by acute cholecystitis (acute infection of the biliary tract), cholelithiasis (gallstones) or biliary ascariasis. The pain accompanied by Cholecystalgia is a kind of paroxysmal colic or a sudden upward drilling pain in the abdominal right upper quadrant. The pain can be so severe that it induces restlessness, an inability to find a comfortable position, emotional upset, nausea, vomiting, spontaneous sweating or rigidity of the limbs.

Point 1

Root of Auricular Vagus (MA-PS)

Location

Root of Auricular Vagus (MA-PS) is an auricular point located at the root of ear, on the juncture between the back of the ear and the mastoid process (See page 203 Auricular point picture).

Method

Acupuncture is used. With the patient in a seated position, stand behind them and push the auricle upward to expose the point. Insert a 1cun needle to a depth of 0.5 cun into the bilateral points. Retain the needles for 20 minutes and rotate them every five minutes. An electric-machine can also be applied for 20 minutes with a continuous wave current.

Result

18 cases were treated with this method and the pain relieved in all of the cases within 15 minutes.

Case

Wang xx, female, 26 years old and pregnant (seven months): Presented with right hypochondriac pain, accompanied by vomiting. Her symptoms were not relieved by anticholinergic medications. Her traditional Chinese medicine diagnosis was biliary ascariasis caused by heat and damp. She was treated using the above method and after three sessions, the pain had markedly improved without further need for medications.

Point 2

Dannang (EX-LE 6)

Location

Danang (EX-LE 6) is an extra point is located on the tender spot 1~2cun directly below Yanglingquan (GB 34) (See Fig. 1-8).

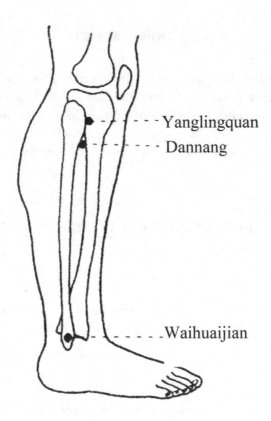

— Yanglingquan

— Dannang

— Waihuaijian

Fig. 1-8 Dannang (EX-LE 6)

Method

Acupuncture is used. Locate the point on both sides while the patient is either seated or lying supine. Insert a 2cun needle perpendicularly and to a depth of 1.5cun into each point. Then, rotate the needles until the patient can feel a Qi sensation travel up along their leg and their abdominal pain decreases. Retain the needles for 20 minutes, If the pain recurs, repeat manipulation every five minutes.

Result

43 cases were treated with this method: the pain stopped in 28 cases; the pain decreased in intensity in 12 cases; and remained the same in two cases.

1.24 Renal colic

Renal colic is usually caused by urinary calculus (kidney stones). The main clinical manifestations include sudden attacks of paroxysmal, lacerating pain over the renal region, which radiates to the external genitalia and medial aspect of the thigh. The pain can last from several minutes to several hours and is accompanied by a pale complexion, cold sweating, nausea and vomiting. In severe cases, shock may ensue. Physical examination will reveal percussion tenderness over the kidney region and tenderness at the costovertebral angle.

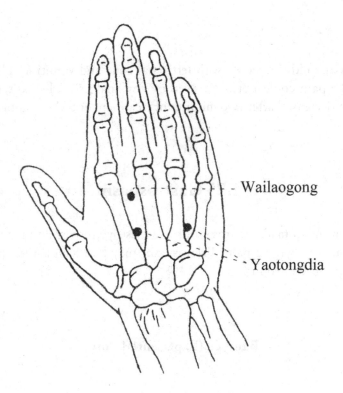

Fig. 1-9 Yaotongdian (EX-UE 7)

Point

Yaotongdian (EX-UE 7)

Location

Yaotongdian (EX-UE 7) is a pair of extra points located on the dorsum of each hand, between the 1st and 2nd and between the 3rd and 4th metacarpal bones and at the midpoint between the dorsal crease of the wrist and metacarpophalangeal joint (See Fig. 1-9).

Method

Acupuncture is used. Locate the points on the affected side and insert a 1cun needle perpendicularly and to a depth of 0.5cun. Rotate the needles strongly using a reducing method until the patient can feel a qi sensation and their pain ceases. Retain the needles for 20 minutes. If pain recurs, repeat manipulation every 5-10 minutes.

Result

21 cases were treated with this method, of which all experienced some pain relief: 17 cases had relief after 3-5 minutes; four cases after 5-10 minutes of treatment; and in two cases their pain came back within 3-6 hours, so the procedure was repeated again and the pain was finally relieved.

Case

Chen xx, male, 30 years old: Presented with left renal colic and vomiting. His X-ray film showed a left renal stone. The pain could not be relieved by any analgesic. He was treated with the above method and his pain decreased after two minutes of treatment and was completely relieved after 10 minutes.

1.25 Gastrospasm

Gastrospasm is a form of stomach neurosis and includes pylorospasm and cardiospasm. The main clinical manifestation is epigastric pain. Pylorospasm may be accompanied by severe pain in the epigastrium, cardiospasm and vomiting.

Point

Banmen (Experiential Point)

Location

Banmen (experiential point) is located on the palmar aspect of the hand at the middle of the 1st metacarpal bone, slightly on the ulnar side of palm (confirm location by local tenderness). (See Fig. 1-10)

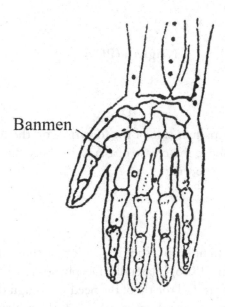

Fig. 1-10 Banmen (Experiential Point)

Method

Acupuncture is used. Select the point on both sides and perpendicularly insert a 1.5 cun needle to a depth of 0.5~1.0 cun. Manipulate the needle strongly with a reducing method until the patient can feel a Qi sensation traveling up their arm and their abdominal pain decreases. Retain the needles for 20~30 minutes. If the pain recurs, repeat needle manipulation every 5~10 minutes.

Result

30 cases were treated with this method, and the pain had markedly decreased in all cases after one treatment.

Case

Shu xx, female, 32 years old: Presented with epigastric pain accompanied by restlessness and sweating after exposure to cold. She was diagnosed with gastrospasm and was treated with the above method. The patient noted pain relief within five minutes, but the needle was retained for an additional 20 minutes for optimum effect.

1.26 Acute Abdominal Pain

Acute abdominal pain is a common clinical symptom. It is caused by functional changes of the internal organs, such as acute gastritis, acute gastroenteritis, spasm of the stomach and/or intestine, biliary ascariasis, acute cholecystitis, acute pancreatitis, acute appendicitis, acute urocystitis and dysmenorrhea. The clinical manifestation is severe abdominal pain.

Point 1

Neiguan (PC 6)

Location

Neiguan (PC 6) is located on the palmar side of the forearm - on the line connecting Quze (PC 3) and Daling (PC 7) - and 2cun above the crease of the wrist, between the tendons of long palmar muscle and radial flexor muscle of the wrist.

Method

Acupuncture is used. Have the patient lie in a supine position, with both knees bent and in a relaxed position. Locate the point Neiguan (PC 6) bilaterally. Deeply insert a 1.5cun needle into each point, towards Waiguan (SJ 5) until you can feel the tip of the needle through the skin on the dorsal (radial) side of the forearm. Have the patient take deep breaths. Ask the patient to hold their breath while the needle is rotated every five minutes for 20~30 minutes. *{Waiguan (SJ 5) is located 2 cun above the transverse crease of dorsum of wrist between the radius and the ulna.}*

Result

200 cases were treated with this method: 119 cases had complete remission; 34 cases markedly improved; 26 cases partially improved and 21 cases did not respond. In 71 % of the improved cases, the pain disappeared after 10 minutes.

Case

Gao xx, male, 19 year-old soldier: Presented with acute abdominal pain that was unresponsive to anticholinergics. He was diagnosed with acute bacillary dysentery and after treatment with the above method. The pain disappeared within five minutes. After seven sessions, the pain had completely relieved.

Discussion

Neiguan (PC 6) is one of the five general points, which can be used to treat all type of chest and abdominal pain. The point Neiguan (PC 6) promotes Yang Qi of all the abdominal organs, thus regulating visceral muscle movement.

Point 2

Zusanli (ST 36)

Location

Zusanli (ST 36) is located on the anterior-lateral side of the leg, 3cun below Dubi (ST 35) and one finger breadth (middle finger) from the anterior crest of the tibia.

Method

Point injection is used. Mix 50mg of phenergan with 0.5mg of atrapine in one syringe. Inject 1/2 the amount into each bilateral point, at a depth of 1.5cm.

Result

77 cases were treated with this method and all had pain relief, although the duration of manipulation varied: six cases required one minute of manipulation; 54 cases required 1-5 minutes; eight cases required 6-10 minutes; another eight cases required 11-20 minutes; and one case required more than two minutes of manipulation.

Discussion

1. The point Zusanli (ST 36) is used for severe cases not responding to needling of the point Neiguan (PC 6).

2. Zusanli (ST 36) is on a dermatome controlled by the L5 nerve, which is responsible for visceral muscle movement.

1.27 Toothache

Toothache is a common symptom within stomatopathy, and can be due to pulpitis, dental caries and periodentitis. Toothache is often aggravated by application of either cold or heat, and is more common of a complaint in children and the elderly with weak physical constitutions.

Point 1

Yatongling (Experiential Point)

Location

Yatongling (experiential point) is located on the palmar aspect of hand, between the 3rd and 4th metacarpal bones, about 5cun proximal to the crease between the metacarpal bone and the phalanges. The exact location depends on local tenderness (See Fig. 1-11).

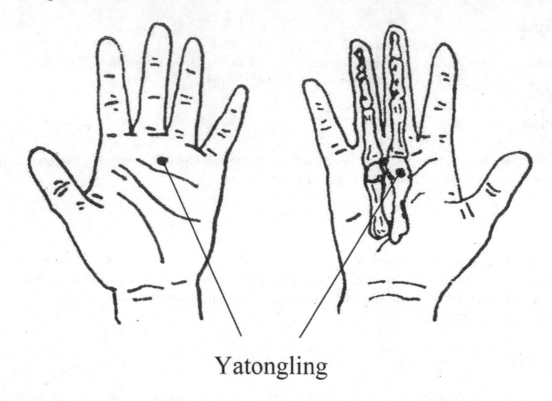

Yatongling

Fig. 1-11 Yatongling (Experiential Point)

Method

Acupuncture is used. Select the point on the affected side. Insert a 1cun needle to a depth of 0.5cun and rotate it using a reducing method until the patient can feel a Qi sensation and the tooth pain improves. Retain the needle for 20 minutes, If the pain recurs, repeat manipulation every five minutes.

Result

112 cases of toothache were all treated for one session: 82 cases had no more pain; 28 cases showed slight improvement; and two cases had no effect.

Point 2

Yemen (SJ 2)

Location

Yemen (SJ 2) is located on the dorsum of the hand, between the 4th and 5th fingers, at the junction of the red and white skin, proximal to the margin of the web.

Method

Acupuncture is used. Select the point on the affected side and insert one cun needle to a depth of 1cun. Rotate using a reducing method until the patient can feel a Qi sensation and their tooth pain improves. Retain the needle for 50 minutes, and if the pain recurs repeat manipulation every 5~10 minutes.

Result

385 cases were treated with this method: 303 showed marked improvement and eight cases did not improve.

Chapter II Internal Diseases

2.1 Arrhythmia

Any abnormality in heart rate, rhythm and cardiac conduction is called arrhythmia and can further be classified as tachycardia, bradycardia and irregular heart beat. Arrhythmia belongs to the categories of "palpitation" and "severe palpitation" in traditional Chinese medicine.

Point

Neiguan (PC 6)

Location

Neiguan (PC 6) is located on the palmar side of the forearm and on the line connecting Quzi (PC 3) and Daling (PC 7), 2 cun above the crease of the wrist, between the tendons of the long palmar muscle and the radial flexor muscle of the wrist.

Method

Acupuncture is used. Locate the points bilaterally and insert a needle 1~1.5cun deep, directed towards to Waiguan (SJ 5). Rotate and lift the needle to manipulate, until the patient can feel a Qi sensation. In elderly patients with chronic arrhythmia, use a reinforcing method. Retain the needles for 15~30 minutes. If the patient is young and also a new case, use the reducing method more strongly and leave the needles for five minutes. Repeat the treatment every day.

Result

84 cases were treated with this method: 14 cases completely resolved; 20 cases markedly improved; 44 cases slightly improved; and six cases had no result.

Case

Wang xx, female, 45 years old: Presented with arrhythmia, palpitation, and chest pain after a family argument. Her heart rate was 180 beats per minute, and an ECG showed frequent premature ventricular beats. She was diagnosed with arrhythmia. After treatment with the above method (and after feeling the Qi sensation for one minute), the patient's breathing and heartbeats were normal in rate and rhythm.

Discussion

1. The point Neiguan (PC 6) belongs to pericardium meridian, and this point is especially used for heart rate regulation. It functions in two ways: the point can be used to decrease fast heart rates, and increase slow heart rates.

2. The point Waiguan (SJ 5) can be used to support the functions of Neiguan (PC 6), and is why the direction of acupuncture needle is towards Waiguan (SJ 5).

2.2 Coronary Atherosclerotic Cardiopathy

Coronary Atherosclerotic Cardiopathy, "coronary heart disease" for short, is due to myocardial ischemia resulting from angiostenosis caused by coronary atherosclerosis. The main clinical manifestations are angina pectoris, myocardial infarction, and myocardial sclerosis. The disease pertains to the TCM categories of "obstruction of Qi in the chest," "angina pectoris" and "precordial pain with cold limbs."

Point

Neiguan (PC 6)

Location

Neiguan (PC 6) is located on the palmar side of the forearm and on the connecting Quzi (PC 3) and Daling (PC 7), 2 cun above the crease of the wrist, between the tendons of the long palmar muscle and the radial flexor muscle of the wrist.

Methods

1. Acupuncture is used. Insert a 2cun needle into each Neiguan (PC 6) point bilaterally to a depth of 1.0 cun and angled towards Weiguan (SJ 5). Rotate the needles quickly for two minutes until the patient can feel a Qi sensation traveling to their elbow, shoulder and heart. If the Qi sensation is local to the point only, press your finger along the pericardium meridian to allow for the Qi sensation to move up. If the Qi sensation still does not flow up to the chest area, stop for five minutes and try again. This time, the needle obliquely towards the heart. Once the patient can feel the correct Qi sensation, retain the needles for 30 minutes. Repeat daily, and one course is equal to 10 sessions.

2. Acupressure is used (the patient can do this on their own). Using the tip of the thumb, press or rub for Neiguan (PC 6) for 10 minutes, 1–2 times daily.

Results

1. 36 cases were treated with the first method: 16 cases presented as an excess type with chest pain and palpitations, and all 16 completely resolved; 20 cases presented as a deficiency type with chest pain only, wherein 18 cases completely resolved and two cases showed no improvement.

2. 20 cases were treated with the second method for two courses: 18 cases had improved and two cases showed no effect.

Cases

1. Pu xx, female, 35 years old: Presented with paroxysmal pain on the left side of her chest for nine days, with the pain radiating to left shoulder and back for the past four days. An ECG showed frequent ventricular premature beats and she was diagnosed with coronary heart disease. She felt severe palpitations, pain and fullness in chest, and had a pale face. She was treated with the first method, and was markedly improved after 20 minutes.

2. Yang xx, male, 51 year-old, officer: Presented with hypertension and coronary heart disease for many years. An ECG showed coronary ischemia. The patient experienced chest pain, a pale face and excessive sweating. After one treatment with the second method, his symptoms improved. Treatment was continued two more times, after which his condition resolved.

Discussion

In severe and acute cases use the first acupuncture method. In mild and chronic case use the second acupressure method.

2.3 Hypertension

Hypertension may be divided into two types: essential hypertension and secondary hypertension. This section will only address protocols for essential hypertension, which is a chronic, systemic vascular disease characterized by rising arterial pressure (especially diastolic pressure), to more than 12.6kPa (95 mmHg). In its early stages, there are symptoms of dizziness, headache, palpitation, insomnia, tinnitus, dysphoria, and lassitude. In later stages, organs such as the heart, brain, kidneys and others may be involved. Essential hypertension belongs to the categories of "dizziness" and "headache" in traditional Chinese medicine.

Point

Shenque (RN 8)

Location

Shenque (RN 8) is located on the middle abdomen, at the center of the umbilicus.

Method

Medicated compress is used. Two kinds of herbs are used in the compress: Chuan Xong (Chuanxiong Rhizome, *Rhizoma Ligustici Chuanxiong*) and Wu Zhu Yu (Evodia Fruit, *Fructus Evodiae*). Grind equal amounts of the herbs together and mix into a thick paste with some vinegar. Fill the patient's navel with the paste and cover the umbilicus with a 4cm square plaster. Change the medicated compress after three days. One course is equal to 10 reapplications. Be careful to keep the area dry and do not allow water to get near the plaster.

Result

118 cases were treated with this method: 77.5% had improved blood pressure after one month of treatment, with the total efficacy rate of 82.3%.

Case

Wang xx, male, 45 year-old doctor: Presented with dizziness and headache of three years duration, with a blood pressure of 21.3/13.3 kPa (160/100 mmHg). The patient's ECG was normal and he was diagnosed with type I hypertension. The patient had ceased using all medications for hypertension when he came in for treatment. The above protocol was used and after five days his blood pressure was within normal limits, and his dizziness and headache had disappeared.

Discussion

Shenque (RN 8) belongs to the Ren meridian and is one of the most important points on the body. The herbs chosen can absorb directly into the bloodstream through the umbilicus and have particular indications to reduce hypertension. Therefore, this method is quite effective in treating hypertension.

2.4 Hypotension

Hypotension is a common clinical symptom. Systolic pressure in a healthy adult should fall between 12.0-18.7 kPa (90-140 mmHg), and diastolic pressure between 8.0-12.0 kPa (60-90 mmHg). Hypotension is when systolic pressure falls to less than 12.0 kPa (90mmHg) and diastolic pressure to less than 8.0kPa (60mmHg). Acute hypotension can manifest in coma and/or shock, and chronic hypotension may have no accompanying symptoms or may include dizziness, giddiness or asthenia.

Point

Xiaergen (MA-PS)

Location

Xiaergen (MA-PS) is an auricular point located at the lower edge of the root of ear (See page 203 Auricular point picture).

Method

Auricular acupuncture is used. Using press needles or ear seeds, place them on the points bilaterally. Press the needle or seeds 2-3 times every day for a duration of 15 minutes each time. After 3-4 days remove the device and replace with a new one. One course of treatment is one month.

Result

49 cases ware treated with this method: All cases completely resolved to a normal blood pressure after three to seven treatments.

Case

Zhang xx, male, 60 years old: Presented with a blood pressure of 90/60 mmHg for the past six months. Accompanying symptoms included dizziness and restlessness. The diagnosis was hypotension from a deficiency of Qi and blood. After two treatments with the above method, his blood pressure elevated to 130/85 mmHg. After continuing another month of treatment, the blood pressure had stabilized.

2.5 Common Cold

The common cold is an acute viral or bacterial inflammation of the upper respiratory tract. Clinically, it manifests as nasal obstruction, runny nose, sneezing, sore throat and a hoarse voice, among others. The common cold may or may not be accompanied by a low fever, lassitude, headache, and/or soreness and pain of the limbs.

Point 1

Fengchi (GB 20)

Location

Fengchi (GB 20) is located on the nape of the neck below the occipital bone, level with Fengfu (DU 16) and in the depression between the upper ends of sternocleidomastoid and trapezius muscles.

Method

Acupuncture is used. Locate the points bilaterally. Insert a 1.5cun needle to a depth of 1cun into each point, directing them both toward the tip of the nose. Use a reducing manipulation until the patient can feel a qi sensation. Retain the needles for 20 minutes. Repeat daily for 3-5 days.

Result

50 cases were treated with this method: The total efficacy rates were 56, 63.5% and 65% improvement within two, four and six days respectively. The efficacy rates of improving headache, cough, runny nose and nasal obstruction were 92%, 29%, 70% and 60%.

Case

Zhang xx, male, 50 year-old officer: Presented with a common cold including headache, cough and runny nose. After three treatments, all of the symptoms disappeared.

Point 2

Dazhui (DU 14)

Location

Dazhui (DU 14) is located on the posterior midline of the nape of the neck, in the depression below the 7th cervical vertebra.

Method

Acupuncture and cupping are used. Insert a 1.5cun needle obliquely toward the head and to a depth of 1cun. Use a reducing manipulation until patient can feel a Qi sensation in the local area, then apply a vacuum-sealed cup for 15 minutes. Repeat every day for 2-3 days.

Result

73 cases were treated with this method and all of the cases improved. Most of the cases required only one treatment, and the rest resolved after 2-3 treatments.

Case

Ma xx, male, 26 year-old worker: Presented with a common cold contracted after exposure to cold and wind after bathing. His symptoms included dizziness, nausea and vomiting. Upon examination, a pale face, sweating, cold legs and arms and a fever were also apparent. After treatment with the above method, his temperature normalized and his symptoms improved.

Discussion

1. The Du meridian controls the six Yang meridians. The common cold with fever is considered a Yang excess condition. The point Dazhui (DU 14) can regulate Yang Qi.

2. The first point Fengchi (GB 20) is best used to treat a common cold without fever and Dazhui (DU 14) is best used when a fever is present.

2.6 Bronchitis

Bronchitis includes both acute bronchitis and chronic bronchitis. Acute bronchitis is an acute inflammation of the trachea or bronchi, caused by a bacterium, virus, physical or chemical irritation. At the onset, it usually has similar symptoms as an infection of the upper respiratory tract, such as fever, aversion to cold, general aching, and cough (as the main symptom). In the beginning the cough tends to be nonproductive, then gradually becomes a productive cough with slight sticky or thin sputum after 1-2 days. After that, purulent, or white and sticky, sputum presents. The course of the disease seldom goes beyond one month.

Chronic bronchitis refers to a chronic inflammation of the bronchial mucosa and tissues around it. Its etiology is associated with viral, bacterium, physical or chemical irritation, immune state, functional nerve disturbance and other factors. The main clinical manifestations are cough with expectoration, and/or accompanied by dyspnea. To be classified as chronic bronchitis, the symptoms must last for at least three months annually, and for more than two consecutive years.

Point

Tiantu (RN 22)

Location

Tiantu (RN 22) is located on the anterior midline of the neck, at the center of suprasternal fossa.

Method

1. Acupuncture is used. The patient should be seated with the back of their head supported. Using a 2 cun needle, first insert it perpendicularly 0.2cun, then rotate the insertion vertically and insert to a depth of 1.5 cun, with the needle tip angled downward (along the posterior aspect of the sternum). Slightly manipulate the needle by rotating it until patient can feel a Qi sensation with local distension and heaviness, then remove. Repeat 1-2 times daily.

2. Point injection is used. Have the patient lie supine, with a pillow under their neck. Using a 5ml syringe, place 1ml of a 10% glucose solution, 1ml of vitamin B1 and 1ml of vitamin B12. Insert the needle obliquely, at about a 40°angle downward to a depth of 3-4cm. Once

the patient can feel a Qi sensation in their chest, including distension and heaviness, push 1/2 the amount of liquid in. Repeat every-other day for about 4-5 times.

Results

1. 50 cases treated with the first method: Acute cases completely resolved after 1-2 treatments and chronic cases required 5-7 treatments for improvement.

2. 800 cases were treated 1-2 times with the second method: 320 cases completely resolved; 400 cases improved and 80 cases had no effect.

Case

Huang xx, male, 42 years old: Presented with cough and chronic bronchitis for two years, which recurred every winter. He took medications, but they had no effect. An X-ray showed increased bronchio-vascular shadows. After one treatment, his cough and sore throat was alleviated and after three treatments, his symptoms markedly improved.

Discussion

1. The first method is for acute and new diseases, whereas the second method is more for chronic disease.

2. The point Tianshu (RN 22) should be used carefully, do not inject more than 2ml of the solution at one time.

2.7 Bronchial Asthma

Bronchial asthma is an allergic disease that presents with repeated attacks. Different antigens, such as pollen, dust, fish, shrimp, fur, and others usually cause the attacks. Pathological characteristics include bronchospasm, muscular edema, and bronchial obstruction due to hypersecretion of fluids. The main clinical manifestation is repeated paroxysmal attacks of expiratory dyspnea with wheezing. The disease belongs to the category of "asthma with wheezing" in traditional Chinese medicine.

Point 1

Danzhong (RN 17)

Location

Danzhong (RN 17) is located on the chest and on the anterior midline, level with the 4th intercostal space and at the midpoint of the line connecting both nipples.

Methods

1. Acupuncture is used. Insert a 2 cun needle horizontally (directing the tip down) to a depth of 1.5cun. Apply a reducing method with rotation until patient can feel a Qi sensation. Retain the needle for 30 minutes. Repeat daily for 10 days.

2. Three–edged needling and cupping therapy are used. Sterilize the local area around the point with a 75% alcohol solution. Use a three-edged needle to induce a little bleeding at the point. Raise and fold skin around the area with the left hand, then apply direct pressure 1~2 times quickly with right hand. For 2~3 minutes, press the area using the aforementioned method to allow for more blood to surface. Then, apply a cup, which will result in even more blood flow. Retain the cup for 15 minutes. The desired amount of blood should total 2~3ml. Repeat every other day for five treatments.

3. Catgut embedding therapy is used. Using a surgical needle, slice around the point at a distance of 1cm from inside to outside. Apply the surgical suture bilateral tips and cover with a plaster. Leave it for two weeks. There is no need to repeat.

Results

1. 35 cases were treated with the first method: 19 cases completely resolved; 11 cases markedly improved; 14 cases slightly improved; and one case showed no result.

2. 13 cases were treated with the second method: nine cases completely resolved and four cases slightly improved.

3. 50 cases were treated with the third method: 35 cases completely resolved; three cases markedly improved; eight cases slightly improved; and four cases showed no effect.

Cases

1. Ding xx, male, 24 year-old worker: Presented with asthma of seven-years duration. The symptoms increased in the winter and autumn, occurring for 5-7 hours at a time, and continuing from days to months. His symptoms included difficulty breathing, fullness in the chest, restlessness and sweating. He had taken many western medications for a long time. After 12 treatments with the first method, his condition had completely resolved.

2. Patient, female, 15 years old: Presented with a common cold since the age of 12. Since then, she has had a cough and asthma, which worsened in poor air quality. After three treatments with the second method, she her symptoms completely resolved.

3. Xong xx, female, 14 year-old student: Presented with a common cold for the past seven years, which then lead to asthma. Presently, her symptoms have worsened. After one treatment with the third method she was completely cured.

Point 2

Dingchuan (EX-B 1)

Location

Dingchuan (EX-B 1) is located on the back of the neck, below the spinous process of the 7th cervical vertebra and 0.5 cun lateral to the posterior midline (See Fig. 2-1)

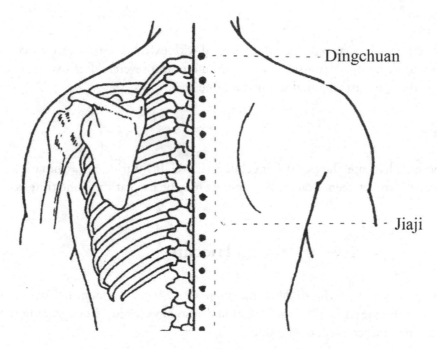

Fig. 2-1 Dingchuan (EX-B 1)

Methods

1. Electrical-acupuncture is used. Locate Dingchuan (EX-B1) bilaterally. Perpendicularly insert a 1.5cun needle to a depth of 1cun, until the patient can feel a Qi sensation in the local area and in the front of their chest. Manipulate with a reducing method during an asthma attack and with a reinforcing method in between attacks. Apply an electric machine at a continuous frequency for 20 minutes. Repeat daily for 10 days.

2. Point injection is used. Select the points bilaterally. Divide 10mg verapamil into a dose of 5mg for each point. Insert the needle to a depth of about 1.5cun, then injecting the liquid after aspiration. Repeat every other day. One course equals 10 treatments.

Results

1. 197 cases were treated with the first method for 1~2 courses: 105 cases completely resolved; 64 cases markedly improved; and 28 cases slightly improved.

2. 40 cases were treated with the second method for 2~9 treatments: 15 cases completely resolved; 12 cases markedly improved; six cases slightly improved; and seven cases had no effect. The total efficacy rate was 82.5%.

Cases

1. Zhang xx, male, 53 year-old, officer: Presented with asthma of ten years. For the past three years, his attacks combined with a common cold every time, lasting about two months. He was treated with the second method and after three injections, his symptoms resolved for 12 years.

2. Gou xx, male, 14 year-old student: Presented with extrinsic asthma after a common cold for three-year duration. His asthma was continuous and severe. After two treatments with the first method, his asthma had stopped for one year.

Discussion

It is more successful to use the point Dingchuan (EX-U 14) during an asthma attack and to use Tanzhong (RN 17) in between attacks. Both points may be used at the same time, as well.

2.8 Hiccup

Hiccup refers to a cramp in the diaphragm, often seen after an abdominal operation or in later stages of a serious disease. A healthy individual may also have hiccup from gulping too much air or consuming too much uncooked, cold food.

Point

Yifeng (SJ 17)

Location

Yifeng (SJ 17) is located posterior to the ear lobe, in the depression between the mastoid process and the mandibular angle.

Methods

1. Acupressure is used. With the patient seated and the practitioner standing behind the patient, place the tips of both index fingers on bilateral Yifeng (SJ 17). Apply simultaneous acupressure, directing the pressure to the opposite point. Have the patient take a deep inhale and hold then hold their breath for as long as possible while applying the acupressure. If the hiccup does not stop after the first round, repeat for 2~3 treatments.

2. Acupuncture is used. Repeat the protocol from method one, using needles instead of acupressure. Insert each needle to a depth of 1cun and rotate once, until patient can feel a Qi sensation. Retain the needles for 30 minutes.

Results

1. 32 mild cases were treated with the first method: 18 cases resolved after first treatment; six cases resolved after the second treatment; five cases resolved after the third treatment; and three cases resolved after the fourth treatment.

2. 126 severe cases of hiccup were treated with the second method: 106 cases obtained complete resolution and 20 cases showed no result.

Cases

1. Liu xx, male, 21 years old: Presented with frequent hiccup after meals, with an inability to sleep. The patient began to self-apply the acupressure technique when the hiccups occurred and his symptoms immediately improved.

2. Wang xx, male, 29 years old: Presented with continuous hiccup for three days. The patient's symptoms increased after meals and he was unable to sleep. Western medications offered no relief. After treatment with the second method, his symptoms resolved completely after three treatments.

Discussion

1. The first method (acupressure) is best suited for mild and acute cases, whereas the second method (acupuncture) is best for the treatment of severe and chronic hiccup.

2. The first method can be used at home to treat hiccup, and is easily administered by the patient themselves or a relative.

3. Having the patient deep breathe during treatment is of utmost importance in efficacy.

2.9 Chronic Gastritis

Chronic gastritis is a nonspecific inflammation of the gastric mucosa. It may be divided into superficial, atrophic and hypertrophic stages, according to the pathogenic process. Main clinical manifestations include epigastric pain, indigestion, anorexia, and others. Chronic gastritis pertains to the category of "epigastric pain" in traditional Chinese medicine.

Point

Zhongwan (RN 12)

Location

Zhongwan (RN 12) is located on the upper abdomen and on the anterior midline, 4cun above the center of umbilicus.

Method

Acupuncture and moxibustion are used. Perpendicularly insert a 2cun needle to a depth of 1.5 cun. Thrust and rotate using a reinforcing method. Once the patient can feel a Qi sensation around the epigastrium, apply moxa to the handle of the needle. Ignite the moxa and let it burn completely. Repeat for a total of three rounds. Repeat daily for up to 10 days.

Result

154 cases were treated with this method: 151 cases with chronic gastritis improved, and cases with chronic gastritis accompanied by cancer or ulcer showed no effect. The total efficacy rate was 98.1%.

Case

Wang xx, male, 58 years old: Presented with pain in his epigastrium for 10 years. The pain was aggravated six months ago and has resulted in a poor appetite and weight loss. Examination by X-ray showed gastritis. After treatment with this method, his symptoms alleviated and his appetite improved after seven treatments. The treatment was continued for an additional seven times every other day, resulting in marked improvement.

Discussion

1. It is necessary to place a piece of paper with a small hole in the center over the skin surrounding the needle before applying moxibustion, so that the moxa will not hurt or burn the patient if some ash falls off.

2. This method is better for chronic stomach pain of the deficiency cold type.

2.10 Vomiting

Vomiting refers to the casting up of food substances or gastric fluid from the stomach and out through the mouth. Vomiting may be seen in many diseases, such as acute or chronic gastritis, cardiospasm, phylorospasm, cholecystitis, pancreatitis and gastroneurosis.

Point

Zhitu (Experiential Point)

Location

Zhitu (experiential point) is located on the palmar aspect of the hand, 0.5cun below the middle of the wrist crease (See Fig. 2-2).

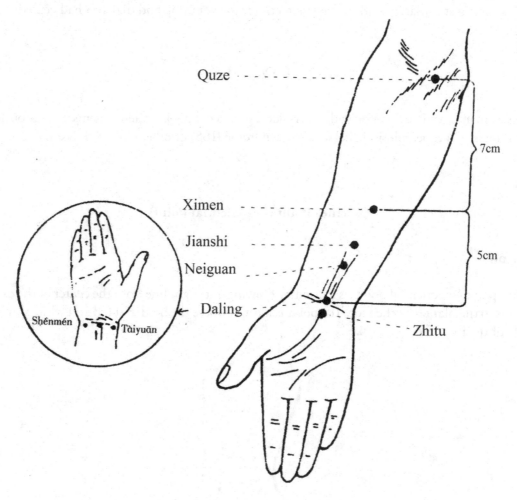

Fig. 2-2 Zhitu (Experiential Point)

Method

Acupuncture is used. Locate bilateral Zhitu (experiential point). Insert a 1cun needle angled obliquely (15°~30°) and toward the tip of the middle finger to a depth of 0.8 cun into each point. Rotate the needles using a reducing method. Once the patient can feel a Qi sensation (numbness/distension in middle finger or hand), retain the needles for 30 minutes. If the vomiting has not stopped, repeat the reducing manipulation every five minutes.

Result

26 cases were treated with this method: 21 cases stopped vomiting after one treatment; five cases ceased after two treatments; and 22 cases did not respond.

Case

Zhang xx, female, one year old: Presented with profuse vomiting and diarrhea for two days. She was vomiting 20 times per night and had bouts of diarrhea at least 10 times per night. Other symptoms included: fever, poor appetite, and an inability to eat or drink anything. After two treatments involving strong stimulation with the above method, the vomiting and diarrhea had ceased.

2.11 Diarrhea

Diarrhea is an increase in defecation with watery, loose or mucoid stool. It often presents in acute or chronic enteritis, intestinal tuberculosis, irritable bowel syndrome (IBS) or other intestinal dysfunction.

Point

Diarrhea Point (Experiential Point)

Location

Diarrhea point (experiential point) is located by drawing a straight line from the center of the external malleolus to the plantar of the foot. The point is located where the border of red and white skin meets the sole of the foot (See Fig. 2-3).

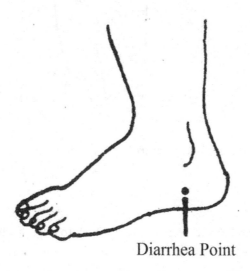

Diarrhea Point

Fig. 2-3 Diarrhea Point (Experiential Point)

Methods

1. Moxabustion is used. Locate the point bilaterally. Ignite a moxa stick and apply the lit end at a distance of 1cun from each point. Switch sides every 15 minutes and repeat 1~2 times daily. One course of treatment is equal to 10 days.

2. Acupuncture is used. Locate the point bilaterally. Insert a 1cun needle perpendicularly to a depth of 0.8cun. Apply a reducing method until the patient can feel a Qi sensation around the local area. Retain the needles for 20 minutes. Repeat daily for five days. If the diarrhea is severe, electrical stimulation may be applied.

Results

1. 120 cases were treated by the first method: 118 cases completely resolved and two cases improved. Of those, 50 cases were treated one time, 59 cases were treated two times, seven cases were treated three times, two cases were treated four times and two cases were treated more than four times.

2. 40 cases were treated with the second method: 85% completely resolved; 7.5% markedly improved; 5% slightly improved; and 2.5% had no effect.

Cases

1. Lin xx, male, 6 months-old: Presented with indigestion, diarrhea (10 bouts daily), restlessness, crying and poor sleep. The infant's stool was watery with white flocculent and a rancid odor. The moxibustion treatment was applied twice, after which, the baby slept well and the diarrhea alleviated. After the third treatment, all symptoms disappeared and the infant was completely cured.

2. Zhuo xx, male, 42 years old: Presented with diarrhea from over-consumption of cold food and drink. The patient complained of loose, watery stool occurring 4-5 times per night. This was also accompanied by pain in the abdomen, intestinal gurgling and tenderness around the umbilicus. The diagnosis was acute diarrhea. After treatment with the second method, the diarrhea stopped and the other symptoms alleviated.

Discussion

The first method (moxibustion) is suitable for children and cases of chronic diarrhea, whereas the second method (acupuncture) is more suitable for adults and acute diarrhea.

2.12 Constipation

Constipation is a condition manifested by prolonged intervals of dry or compacted feces within the intestines, or the desire for immediate bowel movement but with difficulty when defecating. It commonly results in chronic, or habitual, constipation and is due to peristaltic dysfunction or disorders of the rectum or anus (according to Western Medicine).

Point 1

Tianshu (ST 25)

Location

Tianshu (ST 25) are two points located on the middle of the abdomen, 2cun lateral to the center of the umbilicus, on either side.

Methods

1. Acupressure is used. Have the patient lie supine, with knees bent so the abdominal muscles can relax. Using the tip of each index finger, press onto bilateral Tianshu (ST 25) for 10 minutes. Repeat every day. For optimal results, have the patient apply in the morning before getting out of bed. One course is equal to seven days of treatment.

2. Electrical-acupuncture is used. Have the patient lie down supine. Insert 3cun needles into bilateral Tianshu (ST 25). Once the patient can feel a Qi sensation, connect the needles to an electric machine with continuous wave for 30 minutes. Repeat every day.

Results

Eight cases were treated with the second method (electrical acupuncture). In general, by the second day the patients were able to defecate. After seven days of treatment, regular bowel movements were established.

Case

Zhang xx, male, 30 years old: Presented with chronic constipation for one year. He had taken many medications with no avail. He was treated with the second method, and the constipation completely resolved after five treatments.

Point 2

Large Intestine (MA-SC4)

Location

Large intestine (MA-SC4) is an auricular point located in the superior concha of the ear, anterior and superior to the helix crus (See Fig. 19).

Method

Auricular acupuncture is used. Apply press needles or ear seeds onto the points, bilaterally. Cover the press needles with a small adhesive and press three times. Have the patient apply pressure 50 times to each point every day. The pressure should be as strong as the patient can bear. Change the press needles every three days.

Result

80 cases were treated with this method: 72 cases completely resolved; and eight cases did not respond. The needling method described previously was done for an average five treatments before the symptoms improved.

Case

Liu xx, female. 44 years old: Presented with chronic constipation for 17 years, with defecation once every 4-5 days. She was diagnosed with habitual constipation. She was treated by the above auricular method, after five days her stool had softened. After 10 days, she was completely cured.

2.13 Retention of Urine

Retention of urine refers to chronic difficult urination that results in large amounts of urine accumulating in the bladder. Clinically, urinary retention is characterized by a blockage of the urine flow, with distension and fullness in the lower abdomen.

Point

Liniao (Experiential Point)

Location

Liniao (experiential point) is located midway between Qugu (RN 2) and Shenque (RN 8), although it is *not* considered a point on the Ren meridian (See Fig. 2-4).

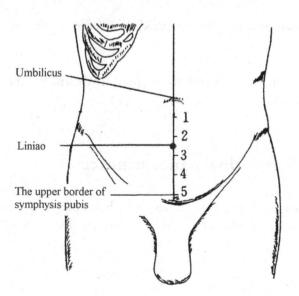

Fig. 2-4 Liniao (Experiential Point)

Methods

1. Acupressure is used. Using the tip of the thumb, start slowly and gently to apply pressure to Liniao (experiential point). Then, begin pressing and rolling for 15 minutes until the patient can feel a desire to urinate. Have the patient continue applying pressure until urination has finished.

2. Acupuncture is used. Insert a 1.5cun needle to a depth of 1cun. Apply a rotating manipulation until the patient can feel a Qi sensation around the local area and has a desire to urinate. Keep the needle in place and repeat manipulation every five minutes until the patient has completed passing urine.

Result

44 cases were treated by both methods and all 40 cases showed good results.

Case

Shun xx, male, 15 year old student: Presented with difficulty urinating after taking a tranquilizer. Other complaints included distension in lower abdomen and restlessness. He was diagnosed with retention of urine. After treatment with the second method, he passed 300 ml of urine within 30 seconds. His urination returned to normal after two hours.

Discussion

1. All of the points between Qugu (RN 2) and Shenque (RN 8) are located on the Ren meridian, which can all be used to treat retention of urine. However, the most effective point is Liniao (experiential point), used in the above protocols.

2. It is important to first use the acupressure method. If no effect is obtained, then proceed to needling.

3. It is best if the patient continues to perform the acupressure treatment on themselves at home, after treatment in clinic.

2.14 Urinary Incontinence

Urinary incontinence refers to involuntary urinary discharge, while a person is conscious/awake. This condition most commonly presents in elderly patients, females or individuals who have survived a traumatic experience.

Point

Ciliao (BL 32)

Location

Ciliao (BL 32) is located on the sacrum, medial and inferior to the posterior-superior iliac spine, just above the 2nd posterior sacral foramen.

Methods

1. Acupuncture is used. Insert a 2 cun needle, bilaterally, and to a depth of 1.5 cun. For deficiency-type urinary incontinence, use a reinforcing manipulation and for excess-type causes use a reducing technique. Once the patient can feel a Qi sensation in their lower abdomen, connect the needles to an electric machine and apply a pulse wave for 30 minutes. Repeat daily.

2. Point injection is used. Inject 2 ml of vitamin B1 with 1ml of 0.9% saline into each point, at a depth of 2cm. Repeat once every other day. One course equals five treatments.

Results

1. 18 cases were treated with the first method for 3-6 treatments: 10 cases completely resolved; seven cases improved; and one case had no effect.

2. 50 cases ware treated with the second method for 1-36 treatments: 37 cases completely resolved; seven cases improved; and six cases showed no effect.

Cases

1. Jiang xx, female, 36 years old: Presented with urinary urgency and frequency for one year. Her symptoms had manifested to involuntary urinary dribbling for the past six months. She was treated with the first method and improved significantly after one treatment. After three treatments, her symptoms completely resolved.

2. Zhu xx, female, three years old: Presented with slow cognitive development, an inability to speak, and involuntary urination and defecation. She was treated with several medications and acupuncture, which had no effect. Her diagnosis was urinary incontinence. After nine treatments with the second method, she could control her urination and defecation, and her cognitive abilities had improved.

Discussion

1. Of the two methods, the first one is best for mild cases of urinary incontinence, and the second is best for more severe cases.

2. It is important to insert the needles at the depression of the sacral foramen, exactly.

2.15 Impotence

Impotence refers to the weakness or inability of the penis to hold an erection during sexual intercourse, and is often characterized by an erection that lasts only for seconds. When impotence presents as the main symptom, it could be due to either sexual neurasthenia or another chronic disease. Etiology and treatment differentiation will be noted throughout this section.

Point

Guanyuan (RN 4)

Location

Guanyuan(RN 4) is located on the anterior midline, 3cun below the umbilicus.

Methods

1. Acupuncture and moxibustion are used. Insert a 3cun needle to a depth of 2-2.5 cun. With a reinforcing method, manipulate the needle until the patient can feel a Qi sensation radiating toward their genitals. Apply a moxa stick to warm the needle, or use up to three direct moxa cones after removing the needle. Repeat daily for up to three treatments.

2. Catgut embedding therapy is used. Sterilize the local area at Guanyuan (RN 4) with a 75% alcohol solution. Using a surgical needle and #00 catgut suture, stitch around the point from top to bottom, with the distance from the inner border to the outside border of the stitch being 1cm. Cut the suture bilaterally and cover it with a bandage. Leave the suture for two weeks. Do not need repeat.

Results

1. 12 cases were treated with the first method for 1-4 treatments: seven cases completely resolved; three cases markedly improved; and three cases slightly improved.

2. 31 cases were treated with the second method for 1-2 treatments: 28 cases completely resolved; and three cases slightly improved.

Cases

1. Wang xx, male, 29 year-old, officer: Presented with impotence of six months duration. He had the ability to initially maintain an erect penis, but it would quickly weaken. He was diagnosed with sexual neurasthenia. After two treatments with the first method, he was markedly improved.

2. Chen xx, male, 42 year-old, officer: Presented with impotence for the past three years. He had tried various medications, with no effect. Upon examination, he displayed normal genitalia.

His diagnosis was sexual neurasthenia. After one treatment with the second method, his symptoms resolved.

Discussion

If the patient does not like to visit the clinic, moxa can be used at home every day over Guanyuan (RN 4) for 30 minutes before sleep.

2.16 Seminal Emission

Seminal emission refers to the involuntary seminal discharge that most often takes place apart from sexual activity or intercourse. Specifically, nocturnal emission happens while dreaming during sleep, while spermatorrhea occurs when the patient is completely clear during sleep (without dreams). Occasional seminal emission in adult males, married or unmarried, is not considered a disorder. For seminal emission caused by prostatitis, neurasthenia, seminal vesiculitis or other disease in western medicine, the differentiation and treatment in this section can be referred to.

Point

Zhongji (RN 3)

Location

Zhongji (RN 3) is located on the anterior midline, 4cun below the umbilicus (See Fig. 31).

Method

Acupuncture and moxibustion are used. Insert a 3 cun needle to a depth of 2~2.5 cun. Stimulate with a reinforcing method until the patient can feel a Qi sensation radiating to their genitals. Apply a moxa stick to warm the needle, or use up to three direct moxa cones after removing the needle. Repeat daily for up to three treatments.

Result

14 cases were treated with this method: 12 cases improved significantly; one case improved slightly; and one case had no effect.

Case

Zheng xx, male, 23 year-old worker: Presented with seminal emission 1~2 times every night for the past six months. Other symptoms included headache, and lower back pain for more than one year. The diagnosis was seminal emission due to deficiency of kidney Yin. He was treated with the above method and was completely cured after eleven treatments. The patient resumed a regular sexual life one year later.

2.17 Facial Paralysis

Peripheral facial paralysis is often caused by an acute non-suppurative inflammation of the facial nerve within the cranial stylomastoid foramen. Clinical manifestations include a sudden onset of numbness or paralysis of the face on the affected side, deviation of the angle of the mouth toward the non-affected side, incomplete closure of the eye on the affected side, a shallow naso-labial groove and overall sluggishness.

Point

Yifeng (ST 17)

Location

Yifeng (SJ 17) is located posterior to the ear lobe, in the depression between the mastoid process and the mandibular angle.

Methods

1. Acupuncture and cupping therapy are used. Insert a 1.5 cun needle into the point on the affected side. Angle the needle toward the other ear and to a depth of 1cun. For an acute case, manipulate with a reducing method and with a reinforcing method for chronic cases until the patient can feel a Qi sensation in local area. Retain the needle for 30 minutes and repeat daily. After removing the needle, apply flash cupping with a pace of 100 quick-cups every five minutes on the affected part of the face (usually the cheek). The cupping should be done quickly and gently so that it does not leave a mark. One course is ten times.

2. Point injection is used. Use a solution of 2 ml vitamin B1 and 1ml vitamin B12, to be injected into the point on the affected side of facial paralysis. Inject 1.5 ml of the mixed solution at a depth of 1cm, directing the insertion toward the other ear. Repeat every other day.

Results

1. 32 cases were treated with the first method for three courses of treatment: 31 cases resolved and one case showed no result.

2. 60 cases were treated with the second method for two courses of treatment: 48 cases completely resolved; 11 cases improved; and one case showed no effect.

Cases

1. Ding xx, male, 26 years old: Presented with the sudden inability to drink water or close his right eyelid one morning. Upon arrival to the clinic, it was noted that his mouth was deviated to the left side and there was a loss of creases in his forehead. The traditional Chinese medicine diagnosis was facial paralysis due to wind and cold. He was treated with the first method and improved after one treatment. His symptoms completely resolved after ten treatments.

2. Zhang xx, female, 53 year-old worker: Presented with left facial paralysis for two years duration, numbness on the left side of her face, facial muscle spasm, and deviation of the angle of her mouth to the right. She went to many doctors, with no improvement. She was diagnosed with left facial paralysis. After three treatments by the second method, she could open her mouth and was able to drink water normally. After four treatments, her symptoms had completely resolved.

Discussion

The first method (acupuncture) is best suited for acute cases, while the second method (point injection) is most effective in chronic cases.

2.18 Facial Spasm

Facial spasm is most common in middle-aged women, and refers to a spasm that comes and goes irregularly on one side of the face. Clinical manifestations initially include intermittent spasms of the orbicular muscles (around the eye). Gradually, the spasm involves other muscles of the face. In severe cases, convulsions of the corner of the mouth ensue. Fatigue, mental stress or physical movement may aggravate the severity of the convulsions or spasm. Some patients may also have headache, and tinnitus. Neurological system examinations will show positive signs and the spasms typically spontaneously stop during sleep.

Point

Houxi (SI 3)

Location

Houxi (SI 3) is located at the junction of the red and white skin along the ulnar border of the hand and at the ulnar end of the distal palmar crease, proximal to the 5th metacarpophalangeal joint when a loose fist is made.

Method

Acupuncture is used. Have the patient in a seated position and locate the point on the affected side. Insert a 1.5cun needle to a depth of 1cun, directing it towards to Hegu (LI 4). Apply a reducing technique by rotating and thrusting, until the patient can feel a Qi sensation. Repeat the manipulation every five minutes, until the patient's threshold. Repeat daily. One course equals three sessions.

Result

Eight cases were treated with this method: one case completely resolved after one treatment; four cases improved after three treatments; and three cases improved after five treatments.

Case

Lui xx, female, 32 year-old assistant: Presented with right-sided facial tics for 15 days duration and paroxysmal right-sided facial muscle spasm that continued for about one hour. She was diagnosed with a facial tic. After treatment with the above method, the spasm had stopped within 30 seconds. The needle was retained for 30 minutes and the patient was completely cured with just one treatment.

2.19 Sequelae to Cerebrovascular Accident

Sequelae to cerebrovascular accident refers to the bundle of symptoms following an acute cerebrovascular disease, including hemiplegia, slurred speech, deviation of the mouth and eye, urinary incontinence, and others. In traditional Chinese medicine, such symptoms pertain to the category of "wind stroke." In this chapter, we will discuss hemiplegia, aphasia, and urinary incontinence as a result of cerebrovascular accident:

<u>Hemiplagia due to Cerebrovscular Accident</u>

Point

Baibui (DU 20)

Location

Baihui (DU 20) is located on the head, 5cun directly above the midpoint of the anterior hairline, at the midpoint of the line connecting the apexes of both ears.

Method

Acupu `ytt5yyncture is used. Insert a 1.5~2 cun needle horizontally under the skin to a depth of 1~1.5 cun, angling the needle to the point Qubin (GB 7) on the affected side. Insert continually through the three sections between the two points Baihui (DU 20) and Qubin (GB 7). Rotate the needle quickly with a frequency of 200 times per minute, continuing for five minutes and resting for five minutes. After 30 minutes repeating this cycle, and remove the needles. Repeat once daily, and one course equals 15 treatments.

Result

500 cases were treated with this method for 1~3 courses: 478 cases were improved and 22 cases had no change.

Case

Sun xx, female, 56 year-old worker: Suffered cerebral thrombosis 14 days prior, and was treated by western medicine with some improvement. She presented with an inability to move the affected side of her body. Her first acupuncture treatment with the above method lasted for 16 hours, after which she could walk about 20 meters with support. After the second treatment, she could walk on her own. Her arm and hand were able to move after three treatments.

Aphasia due to Cerebrovscular Accident

Point

Yumen (Experiential Point)

Location

Yumen (experiential point) is located on the midline of the underside of the tongue, 1cun from the tip of tongue (See Fig. 2-5).

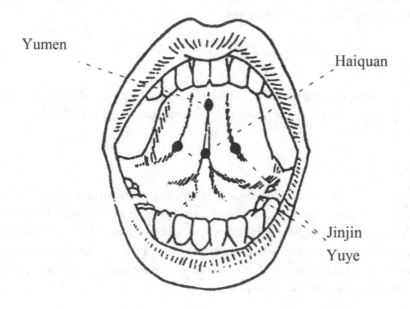

Yumen

Haiquan

Jinjin
Yuye

Fig. 2-5 Yumen (Experiential Point)

Method

Acupuncture is used. Have the patient seated or lying down, with the mouth open. The left hand of the practitioner should be gloved and grasping the patients tongue. Using the right hand, insert a 2cun needle horizontally to a depth of 1.5cun and direct it toward the root of tongue. Use an even technique until patient feels a heat sensation in the throat and can say "Ah---". Treat once daily, with one course equal to six treatments. Rest for 3~5 days between each treatment course.

Result

75 cases were treated with this method, and all of the cases improved.

Urinary Incontinence due to Cerebrovascular Accident

Point

Tongtian (BL 7)

Location

Tongtian (BL 7) is located on the head, 4cun directly above the midpoint of the anterior hairline and 1.5cun lateral to the midline.

Method

Acupuncture is used. Insert a 1.5~2cun needle horizontally and to a depth of 1~1.5cun into the points bilaterally. Angle the needles toward the point Luoque (BL 8), and rotate quickly (200 times per minute). Continue rotating for three minutes, then rest five minutes, and then continue three minutes again, alternating for about 30 minutes.

Result

30 cases were treated with this method for 3~10 treatments: 15 cases completely resolved; 10 cases markedly improved; three cases slightly improved; and two cases had no effect.

Case

Li xx, female, 65 years old: Presented with headache and dizziness for one month before the sudden onset of hemiplegia, aphasia, urinary and bowel incontinence and eventually, coma. Her blood pressure was 26.7/16.0 kPa (200/120 mmHg), and a CT scan showed left cerebral hemorrhage. She was treated by western medicine with some improvement, but her urinary incontinence persisted. After one treatment by the above method, she was able to have sensation upon urination and after three treatments she could control her urination.

2.20 Rheumatic Chorea

Rheumatic chorea refers to involuntary movements accompanied by the disturbance of voluntary movement, muscle weakness and emotional instability. Rheumatic chorea may also be known as minor chorea and is mostly seen in children and female adults. It is mainly caused by rheumatic fever. However, factors like scarlet fever, diphtheria, encephalitis and hypothyroidism may also give rise to rheumatic chorea.

Point

The Chorea-Trembling Controlled Area

Location

The chorea-trembling controlled area is located 1.5cun in front of the motor area, and parallel to it (See Fig. 2-6).

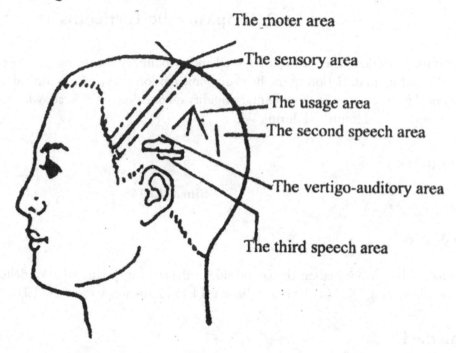

Fig. 2-6 The Chorea-Trembling Controlled Area

Method

Acupuncture is used. Have the patient in a seated position. Insert a 1.5 cun needle to a depth of 1cun and at a 30° angle. Rotate the needle about 150-200 times per minute continuously for three minutes, then rest for two minutes, and so on for three repetitions per session. Repeat daily for ten days (one course). Rest for 2-3 days between each course.

Result

20 cases were treated with this method for one course of treatment. Of that, 13 cases were between 5-10 years old and seven cases were between the ages of 10-20: 14 cases completely resolved; five cases improved; and one case showed no effect.

Case

Ding xx, male, 16 year-old student: Developed pressure within the eyes and visual flashing disturbance for two months. After five days of the aforementioned symptoms, his mouth and right hand began to move involuntary and his head began to involuntary shake to the right and left. Examination showed the patient to be conscious, without a speech problem and with a normal eye exam. The diagnosis was rheumatic chorea. After one treatment, he regained control of moving his mouth and right hand. After five treatments, he could control all movements and after ten treatments his symptoms completely resolved.

2.21 Spasmodic Torticollis

Spasmodic torticollis refers to paroxysmal and involuntary contraction of the cervical muscles of the neck, leading to deviation of the head or clonic tension to one side. Clinical manifestations include cervical muscle spasm and involuntary rigidity on one side of the head, which is often aggravated by nervousness and improved during sleep.

Point

Binao (LI 14)

Location

Binao (LI 14) is located on the lateral side of the arm, at the insertion of deltoid muscle and on the line connecting Quchi (LI 11) and Jiaoyu (LI 15), 7cun above Quchi (LI 11).

Method

Acupuncture is used. Locate the points bilaterally and have the patient find a comfortable seated position. Insert a 2 cun needle obliquely to a depth of 1.5 cun and directed downward (toward the hand). Apply a reducing technique until the patient can feel a Qi sensation radiating to their hand. Retain the needles for 30 minutes.

Result

Four cases were treated with this method and all cases improved.

Case

Liang xx, male, 40 year-old farmer: Presented with a sudden onset of torticollis two months ago, including muscle spasm on the right side of the neck and deviation of the head to the right at an angle of 45°. Each spasm lasted for about 3-5 seconds, with 30 minutes between onset. All spasms occurred while the patient was conscious, and never during sleep. He was diagnosed with spasmodic torticollis. After four treatments with the above method, his symptoms resolved. One year later, the symptoms recurred and the same treatment was given two more times with complete resolution and no recurrence.

2.22 Numbness of the Hand

Numbness of the hand, which is generally caused by cervical spondylopathy, included numbness or pain of the fingers, hands, arms, rigidity of the fingers, difficulty moving the hands, and decreased strength. The symptoms can occur either unilaterally or bilaterally and some cases are accompanied by dizziness, nausea or blurry vision.

Point

Jingbi (Experiential Point)

Location

Jingbi (experiential point) is located above the upper border of the clavicle, on the internal 1/3 and external 2/3 of the external border of the sternocloidal-mastoid muscle (See Fig. 2-7).

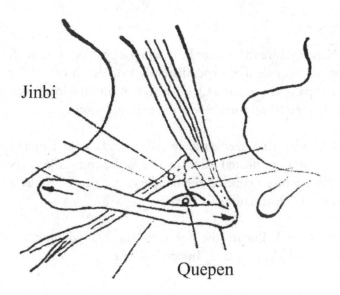

Jinbi

Quepen

Fig. 2-7 Jingbi (Experiential Point)

Method

Acupressure is used. The patient should be seated with the practitioner standing in front of them. Locate the point on the affected side. Steady the patient's shoulder with your left hand while the tip of the thumb on the other hand presses and rolls on the point. First, apply gentle pressure, gradually increasing until the patient can feel an electric sensation radiating down to the affected hand. Continue for about 15 minutes and repeat daily 2~3 times.

Result

200 cases were treated with this method: Most cases improved after 1-2 treatments, with no recurrence.

2.23 Systremma

Systremma refers to a sudden colic spasm of the lateral or bilateral gastrocnemius muscle. It is usually caused by cold and symptoms are alleviated by warmth. Clinical manifestations include pain in the lower leg, difficulty moving, and paroxysmal spasm.

Point

Chengshan (BL 57)

Location

Chengshan (BL 57) is located on the posterior midline of the leg, between Weizhong (BL 40) and Kunlun (BL 60), in a depression formed below the gastrocnemius muscle belly when the leg is stretched or the heel is lifted.

Methods

1. Acupuncture is used. Have the patient lie in a prone position. Locate the point on the affected side and insert a 3 cun needle perpendicularly to a depth of 1.5-2 cun. Apply a reducing method until the patient can feel a Qi sensation around the local area. Retain the needle for 30 minutes and every 10 minutes repeat the manipulation again.

2. Moxibustion with warming needle therapy is used. Have the patient lie in a prone position. Locate the point on the affected side. Insert a 2-3 cun needle perpendicularly to a depth of 1.5-2 cun. Place a moxa cone on the handle of the needle, ignite it and repeat using 2-3 moxa cones in total. Treat daily.

3. Point injection is used. Locate the point on affected side and create a solution of 2ml vitamin B1 with 1ml vitamin B12. Inject 3ml of the solution at a depth of 2cun into the point.

Results

1. 23 cases were treated with the first method: 80% of the cases completely resolved within one session.

2. Nine cases were treated with the second method for 1-3 treatments: seven cases completely resolved and two cases improved.

3. 30 cases were treated with the third method: Most of the cases had alleviated symptoms after one treatment, and the rest improved after 2-3 treatments.

Case

Lui xx. male, 65 years old: Presented with bilateral systremma for five years duration. The symptom was aggravated by cold and resulted in paroxysmal spasm 2-3 times during the night. After three treatments with the first method, his symptoms completely resolved with no recurrence for one year.

Discussion

The fist method is only to be used at the first onset of persistent spasm and pain. In the cases of chronic spasm, use the second or the third method.

2.24 Epilepsy

Epilepsy is defined as a paroxysmal and temporary disturbance of the brain characterized by a loss of consciousness, muscle tics and an overall abnormal sensation, emotion or behavior. Clinical manifestations of the disease vary greatly. Epilepsy can be classified as grand mal, petit mal, rolandic mal or infantile spasms. The grand mal type is characterized by a sudden loss of consciousness, general spasm with apnea, cyanosis and foaming at the mouth, which usually lasts for 1-5 minutes. After such an attack, the patient may fall asleep and become conscious a few hours later. A petit mal is characterized by a sudden, short loss of consciousness without aura, muscle tic or presence of speech or movement interruptions. A petit mal usually persists for 2-10 seconds and the patient will usually return to consciousness rapidly.

Point

Dazhui (DU 14)

Location

Dazhui (DU 14) is located on the posterior midline, in the depression below the 7th cervical vertebra.

Method

Acupuncture is used. The patient should be seated with the neck flexed forward. Insert a 1.5cun needle obliquely to a depth of 1.0cun angled upward (no manipulation). Once the patient feels an electric sensation radiate to their arms, remove the needle. Repeat daily or every other day. One course equals ten treatments and rest for seven days between each course.

Result

95 cases were treated with this method: 24 cases markedly improved with a decrease in frequency and duration of epileptic attacks; 45 cases improved; and 26 cases showed no result.

Case

Zheng xx, female, 12 year-old student: Presented with epilepsy as a result of a head injury since the age of five. Of late, she experienced an epileptic attack 1-2 times daily. She tried taking the western medication Dilantin, with no result. Over the past six months, the frequency of epileptic attacks had increased. An electroencephalogram showed abnormalities and she was diagnosed was epilepsy. She was treated with the above method for seven treatments, after which the frequency of epileptic attacks decreased to once per week, and with a duration of only five minutes. After 25 treatments, the frequency decreased to once every four weeks, and to a duration of two minutes. After 35 treatments, all epileptic attacks had ceased, the patient's electroencephalogram was normal, and all medications were stopped. After five years, the epilepsy was completely gone.

Discussion

Do not manipulate strongly or with deep insertion (to avoid damaging the marrow). The point regulates Qi in all six of the Yang meridians, and can thus regulate brain function.

2.25 Vertigo

Dizziness is the general term for blurred vision and/or vertigo. The former refers to the blurring of vision with darkness appearing in front of the eyes. The latter refers to a subjective feeling that the body or surrounding objects are actually in motion with a difficulty keeping balance. They are always mentioned together since they commonly appear at the same time. Mild dizziness may be stopped instantly by closing the eyes. In severe cases, the patient feels as if they are on a fast-moving train or sailing a boat, which makes it difficult to stand firmly. Such episodes may be accompanied by nausea, vomiting, sweating or fainting. Dizziness may also be seen in other western medical diseases such as auditory vertigo, cerebral arteriosclerosis, hypertension, vertebrobasilar ischemia, anemia, neurasthenia and cerebral conditions where dizziness is the main symptom. Differentiation in treatment for any of the aforementioned conditions will be referred to in this section.

Point

Baihui (DU 20)

Location

Baihui (DU 20) is located on the head, 5cun directly above the midpoint of the anterior hairline and at the midpoint of the line connecting the apexes of both ears.

Methods

1. Acupuncture is used. Have the patient in a seated position. Insert a 1.5cun needle into Baihui (DU 20), directed toward Shishenchong (EX-4). First direct the needle anteriorly, then to the left, then to the right, and finally posteriorly until the patient can feel a Qi sensation at

each turn. Do not remove and reinsert the needle, but rotate at each turn until the patient feels heaviness in their head. Retain the needle for 24 hours.

2. Moxibustion is used. Have the patient seated and remove hair around the local area at Baihui (DU 20). Rub the point with ginger. Take a piece of ginger sliced 0.3cm thick and punch several holes in it with an acupuncture needle. Then, place it on Baihui (DU20) with a moxa cone placed on top of the ginger. Ignite the moxa cone and let it burn until the local skin becomes flush and wet. In general, each treatment will utilize 7-10 moxa cones, repeated once daily. One course is ten days.

Result

22 cases were treated with the first method: 18 cases completely resolved; two cases improved; and two cases had no result. The average treatment number was ten for each case.

Case

Kong xx, female, 52 year-old worker: Presented with right-sided hemiplegia for three years duration, left-sided hemiplegia for one year duration, dizziness, insomnia, difficulty speaking, numbness in the arm, and difficulty moving her hands. The diagnosis was vertigo due to deficiency of Qi and blood. After one treatment with the second method, the patient noted an increase in clarity of her head and eyes. After ten treatments, her symptoms had completely resolved.

Discussion

The two methods can be used for different types of vertigo. The first method (acupuncture) is used in excess types, and the second method (moxibustion) is better for deficiency types. Baihui (DU 20) is a point at which the 12 meridians meet each other. Vertigo is often due to cold and Yang Qi deficiency (deficiency type) or stagnation (excess type), and the point Baihui (DU 20) addresses all such patterns.

2.26 Schizophrenia

Schizophrenia is the most common form of psychosis, yet the etiology is not well understood despite many years of research. In general, genetic and environmental factors are considered to be involved in occurrence of the disorder. Schizophrenia frequently occurs in young adults and the ratio of incidence between males and females is roughly equal. Main characterizations of the disorder include incoherent thinking/speaking, apathy, delusion, and hallucinations (to name a few). Schizophrenia belongs to the category of "manic-depressive psychosis" in traditional Chinese medicine.

Point

Fengfu (DU 16)

Location

Fengfu (DU 16) is located 1cun directly above the midpoint of the posterior hairline, directly below the external occipital protuberance, in the depression between both sides of the trapezius muscles.

Method

Acupuncture is used. Insert a 1.5cun needle perpendicularly and angled toward the tip of the nose to a depth of 1cun. Depending on the characterizations of the disease, use a tonify, reducing or even stimulation (it is not necessary to apply aggressive stimulation). Once the patient can feel a Qi sensation, remove the needle. Repeat the treatment once daily, and ten treatments equals one course.

Result

10 cases were treated with this method for 1-2 courses: all of the cases showed improved symptoms.

Case

Patient, male, 26 years old: Presented with signs of a mental disorder for the past four months, which included emotional depression, apathy, dementia, divagation, muttering to himself, frequent crying or laughing for no apparent reason, caprice, and no desire for food. His tongue had a greasy-white coating, and his pulse was taut and slippery. He was diagnosed with schizophrenia. After being treated with this method for six treatments, all of his symptoms improved.

2.27 Hysteria

Hysteria is a common type of neuroses, and occurs more often in young women. The disease is characterized by delusions of grandeur, volatile mannerisms, and hypersensitivity. Hysteric attacks of are often related to mental imbalance. In this section, psychonosema, aphasia and paralysis are referred to as a result of hysteria.

Psychonosema from Hysteria

Point

Renying (ST 9)

Location

Renying (ST 9) is located on the neck, lateral to the laryngeal protuberance and on the anterior border of sternocleidomastoid muscle (where the pulsation of the common carotid artery is palpable).

Method

Acupuncture is used. Have the patient lie on their back, and place a small pillow under their shoulders so that the anterior surface of the neck is exposed. Locate the point bilaterally and slowly insert a 1cun needle to a depth of about 0.3–0.5 cun. Once the handles of the needles are undulating and the patient can feel a Qi sensation in the form of numbness, distension and/or soreness, retain the needles for 30 minutes. Depending on the case, electrical stimulation may be applied to enhance the therapeutic effect.

Result

148 cases were treated with this method: all of the cases demonstrated good results within one treatment, with an improved functioning of their mental state and clarity of speech.

Case

Patient, female, 30 years old: Presented with sudden and uncontrollable movement of her legs and arms, difficulty speaking, and disorientation. After treatment with the above method, she could walk normally, speak clearly, and all other symptoms disappeared within ten minutes.

Aphasia from Hysteria

Point

Lianquan (RN 23)

Location

Lianquan (RN 23) is located on the neck and on the anterior midline, above the laryngeal protuberance and in the depression above the upper border of hyoid bone.

Method

Acupuncture is used. Have the patient seated with the head slightly tilted back. Insert a 2cun needle obliquely angled upward to a depth of 1.5cun. Once the patient can feel a strong Qi sensation involving local soreness and distension, slightly pull back on the needle, and change direction of insertion to the left Jinjin (EX-HN 12) and to the right Yuye (EX-HN 13). Insert no farther than a depth of 1cun, and stimulate with a rotating method. Simultaneously, instruct the patient to say: "Ah----", "Ba----" or "one, two----". Repeat treatment every day or every other day.

Result

30 cases were treated with this method, all of which resolved eventually: 18 cases resolved in five treatments; seven cases resolved in 12 treatments; and five cases resolved in 13 or more treatments.

Paralysis due to Hysteria

Point

Huantiao (GB 30)

Location

Huantiao (GB 30) is located on the lateral side of the thigh, at the junction of middle third and distal third of the line connecting the prominence of the greater trochanter and the sacral hiatus - when the patient is in a lateral recumbent position with the thigh flexed (See Fig. 37).

Method

Acupuncture is used. Have the patient lie in a lateral recumbent position. Insert a 3cun needle perpendicularly and angled toward the genitals to a depth of 2.5cun. Rotate and lift the needle with a reducing method until the patient can feel the sensation travel down to their feet on the same side. Remove the needle and repeat on the other side. Repeat the bilateral treatment once daily.

Result

41 cases were treated with this method and all cases improved after one treatment.

2.28 Insomnia

Insomnia is a condition that inhibits a person from acquiring normal hours of sleep. It is usually accompanied by dizziness, headache, palpitation and poor memory. However, insomnia may present with different clinical manifestations. In mild cases, it may be difficult to fall into sleep, or dream-disturbed sleep that causes frequent waking, emotional upset and the inability to fall asleep again. In severe cases, a person may be unable to sleep through the whole night.

Point

Zudigenbu (Experiential Point)

Location

Zudigenbu (experiential point) is located at the intersection of the following two lines: 1) From center of interior malleolus to center of exterior malleolus. 2) From the middle toe to the heel (See Fig. 2-8).

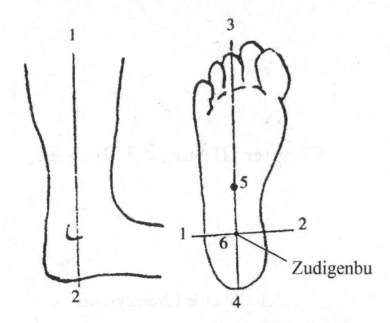

Fig. 2-8 Zudigenbu (Experiential Point)

Method

Acupuncture is used. Select the points bilaterally. Insert a 1cun needle to a depth of 0.5~0.8 cun and apply even stimulation by rotating the needles for 1~2 minutes. Retain the needles for 30 minutes or more and repeat daily. One course is equal to six treatments.

Result

77 cases were treated with this method for 1~4 courses: 60 cases markedly improved (with an ability to sleep 7~8 hours per night, and all secondary-symptoms disappeared); 15 cases slightly improved (with the sleep time extended, and a decrease in secondary symptoms); two cases showed no result.

Case

Liao xx, male, 28 year-old, officer: Presented with insomnia for two years with specific difficulty falling asleep before midnight. Other symptoms included palpitation, dizziness, and asthenia. The symptoms improved after one treatment by the above method. After continuing treatment for one course, the insomnia was cured.

Chapter III Surgical Diseases

3.1 Chronic Cholecystitis

Chronic cholecystitis is a common illness that often requires surgery. More than 90% of recurrent episodes of cholecystitis are associated with the presence of gallstones. Such attacks are often less severe than classical acute cholecystitis, which may resemble peptic ulceration, peptic esophagitis or myocardial ischemia.

Point

Shenque (RN 8)

Location

Shenque (RN 8) is located on the middle abdomen and at the center of the umbilicus.

Method

Moxibustion is used. Have the patient lie down in a supine position. Ignite a moxa stick and hold it 1~2cun above the umbilicus, moving it in small circles until the local area is very warm (as much as the patient can tolerate). Apply for 20 minutes daily.

Result

21 cases were treated with this method: 15 cases completely resolved; four cases slightly improved; and two cases showed no effect.

Case

Guan xx, male, 45 year-old doctor, Presented with chronic cholecystitis as a result of gall stones for many years. His symptoms included distention of the abdomen, nausea, and epigastric pain that radiated to the right shoulder. He had taken Atropine, with no relief and an increase of pain by the next day. His diagnosis was cholecystitis. He was treated with the above method and after two minutes of moxa application, the pain had decreased. After five minutes, the pain disappeared.

Discussion

The smoke of burning moxa contains volatile oils that penetrate through the skin and transfer warmth into the meridian.

3.2 Cholelithiasis

Cholelithiasis is a common surgical disease, which is both caused and affected by cholecystitis. Inflammation and gallstones are usually found simultaneously, so the clinical manifestations are similar to each other. For the most part, gallstones do not produce significant symptoms on their own, but they may lead to: flatulence, biliary colic, acute cholecystitis, chronic cholecystitis and obstructive jaundice (which may further involve intermittent fever, jaundice and upper abdominal pain). Gallbladder empyema from obstruction of the bile duct may also occur, but is uncommon.

Point

Danshu (BL 19)

Location

Danshu (BL19) is located on the mid-back, below the spinous process of the 11th thoracic vertebra, 1.5 cun lateral to the posterior midline.

Method

Acupuncture is used. Have the patient lie down in a prone position. Locate the points bilaterally and insert 1.5 cun needles to a depth of 1cun into each point. Angle the needles obliquely and towards the midline and apply a reducing manipulation. Once the patient can feel a Qi sensation in local area, apply an e-stimulation machine with continuous frequency and strong stimulation. Retain the needles for 40 minutes and repeat the treatment daily.

Result

50 cases were treated with this method: 40 cases completely resolved and one case showed no effect.

Case

Zhuo xx, female, 46 years old: Presented with gallstones for the past five months. Her symptoms included epiggastric pain, paroxysmal colic (radiating toward the right shoulder), vomiting undigested food, fever, chills and a poor appetite. Upon evaluation, the patient's temperature was 39°C and there was tenderness of the right epigastrium. She was diagnosed with cholecystitis. After receiving one treatment by the above method, her pain had decreased by the next day and 0.5g of gallstones was detected in her stool. After the third treatment, one stone passed in her stool with the following measurements: 3.6 × 2 × 1cm and 5.1g in weight. Her symptoms completely resolved after six treatments.

3.3 Biliary Ascariasis

Biliary ascariasis refers to a kind of paroxysmal colic or a sudden upward "drilling" pain of the upper abdomen, caused by an upward movement of ascarid from the intestines into the biliary duct. The pain will cause the patient to turn from side to side in bed, cry, vomit, have excessive sweating, nausea or potentially suffer from rigidity of the limbs (in severe cases). The pain can quickly be relieved and the patient returns to normal once the ascarid has withdrawn from the biliary duct.

Point

Yingxiang (LI 20)

Location

Yingxiang (LI 20) is located in the nasolabial groove, at the level of the midpoint of the lateral border of ala nasi.

Method

Acupuncture is used. Have the patient lie in a supine position. Perpendicularly insert a 1cun needle 0.5cm into each point, then changing direction and angling the needles toward the acupuncture point Sibai (ST 2) at a horizontal insertion. Apply a reducing method. Cut off the handle and place a plaster over the exposed needle. Repeat on the other side and for leave 24 hours. There is no need to repeat this treatment.

Result

22 cases were treated with this method: 13 cases completely resolved (of that, five cases passed ascarids in their stool); six cases slightly improved; and three cases had no change.

Discussion

The point Yingxiang (LI 20) is located on the large intestine meridian, which flows into the stomach meridian. It is the linking of these two meridians that makes the muscle of the gallbladder relax. Therefore, this treatment can decrease pressure and allow the ascarid to withdraw.

3.4 Volvulus

Volvulus refers to a rotated section of the intestine, most often of the small intestine, and can lead to intestinal obstruction. Volvulus is characterized by the following symptoms: abdominal pain, vomiting, abdominal distention, flatulence and difficulty evacuating the bowels. Such symptoms are caused by impeded intestinal transportation function caused by stagnation and obstruction of intestines.

Point

Zhangmen (LR 13)

Location

Zhangmen (LR 13) is located on the lateral side of the abdomen, below the free end of the 11th rib.

Method

Acupuncture is used. Have the patient lie in a supine position. Locate the points bilaterally and insert 1cun needles to a depth of 0.5cun into each point, horizontally. Direct the needles toward the midline and apply a reducing method until patient can feel distension or numbness in the local area. Then, apply an e-stimulation machine with continuous wave frequency and strong stimulation. Retain the needles for 20~60 minutes, and repeat 1~2 times daily.

Result

114 cases were treated with this method: 102 cases completely resolved and were able to pass stools; 12 cases showed no result and needed to undergo surgery. Most of the successful cases received results after 30~60 minutes of treatment.

Case

Song xx, male, 24 year-old worker: Presented with sudden abdominal pain, vomiting, distension, an inability to pass gas or stool, enlarged abdomen, and intestinal ansa around the umbilicus - all of which resulted after beginning work after meal. The diagnosis was volvulus. He was treated with the above method and after seven minutes he was able to pass gas and the pain and distention had decreased. By the second day, all was resolved.

Discussion

The point Zhangmen (LR 13) can also be used for post-operative intestinal paralysis.

3.5 Acute Mastitis

Acute mastitis refers to sudden inflammation of the mammary gland, often caused by bacterial infection. The infection can occur via nipple lacerations or from the retention of milk in breast-feeding women. This condition is most likely to occur 3-4 weeks after childbirth.

Point

Jianjing (GB 21)

Location

Jianjing (GB 21) is located on the shoulder, directly above the nipple, at the midpoint of the line connecting Dazhui (DU 14) and the acromion, at the highest point of the shoulder.

Method

Acupuncture is used. Have the patient seated and locate the point on the affected side. Insert a 1cun needle perpendicularly to a depth of 0.5-0.8cun and apply a reducing method by rotating until the patient feels a sensation of numbness and distension radiating to their shoulder and elbow. Manipulate the needle for 5-10 minutes, then remove. Repeat this procedure two times daily until the symptoms have resolved.

Result

393 cases were treated with this method: 390 cases completely resolved (320 resolved in 1-3 treatments, 50 cases resolved in 3-7 treatments, 13 cases resolved in 7-15 treatments, and one case resolved in more than 15 treatment); three cases had no result.

Case

Yu xx, female, married and a farmer: Presented with a distended and swollen breast for the past five days, accompanied by chills, fever (temperature of 38.9°C), headache, redness of the left breast and a 8 × 9 cm painful engorgement that refused pressure. She was diagnosed with acute mastitis. Her symptoms improved after two treatments with the above method as her temperature reduced to 36.7° C, and the breast pain and swelling had decreased. She received another two treatments, after which, her condition resolved.

Discussion

The point Jinjing (GB 21) is on the foot Shaoyaong meridian, and crosses with the foot Yangming and Yangwei meridians - which all have a close relationship to the breast. Therefore, the point can decrease fire trapped inside the breast and reduce stagnation of blood to treat mastitis.

3.6 Ureterolithiasis

Ureterolithiasis, or urinary calculus, is a common disease of the urinary system and includes kidney, ureter, vesical, and urethral calculi.

Point

Taixi (KI 3)

Location

Taixi (KI 3) is located in the depression between the tip of the medial malleolus and the Achilles tendon.

Method

Acupuncture is used. Have the patient lie in a comfortable position. Locate the points bilaterally. Insert a 1cun needle to a depth of 0.5 cun into each point, angling the needles toward Kunlun (BL 60). Apply a reducing method with strong stimulation until the patient can feel numbness and distension radiating to their feet. Retain the needles for 30-90 minutes and repeat once daily.

Result

23 cases were treated with this method for 1-3 treatment: 18 cases significantly improved as they all experienced cessation of pain in local area, and of that six were able to pass stones in their urine; five cases slightly improved.

Case

Yan xx, male, 54 years old: Presented with pain of the left lumbar region, colic pain of the left lower abdomen, nausea, vomiting, frequent micturition and urinary urgency. Upon examination, the patient was pale in color, had marked tenderness of the left lower abdomen, a positive test for blood cells in the urine, and one visible 0.8 × 0.6 cm stone upon X-Ray. The diagnosis was left urethral calculi. He was treated with the above method and his pain decreased within one minute after the needle was inserted. After one follow-up treatment the next day, his condition had completely resolved.

3.7 Chronic Prostatitis

Chronic prostatitis is a very common disorder of the urinary system, affecting young and middle-aged males. It is usually a secondary infection to acute prostatitis or posterior urethritis. Sometimes, chronic prostatitis may also be a secondary infection to an upper respiratory tract infection or mouth cavity. The most common pathogens include staphylococcus, streptococcus and colibacillus. Excessive consumption of alcohol, injury to the perineum or excessive sexual intercourse is possible causative factors.

Point

Shenque (RN 8)

Location

Shenque (RN 8) is located on the abdomen, at the center of the umbilicus.

Method

Medicated compress therapy is used. Have the patient lie in a supine position. Gather the following herbs: 0.15g of Musk (Moschus) and 7.9g of White Pepper. Mix the two herbs to make a combined powder. Clean the umbilicus with a 75% alcohol solution and place one spoonful of the mixed powder into the umbilicus. Cover the area with cotton and then a plaster. Change the dressing and compress after seven days. Four cycles equals one course of treatment, and it usually takes six courses to get the best result.

Result

11 cases were treated with this method (all with a long history of chronic prostatitis ranging from three months to six years): six cases completely resolved; three cases improved; and two cases showed no result.

Case

Huang xx, male, 50 year-old Officer: Presented with a sensation of heat and pain in the perineum, difficult urination, pain of the urethra and a swollen prostate (upon palpation). The diagnosis was chronic prostatitis. After three courses of treatment by the above method, his symptoms disappeared and the condition resolved.

3.8 Hemorrhoids

Hemorrhoid(s) present when veins in the rectum and anus become swollen and/or twisted. In general, hemorrhoids present as fleshy prominences found at the internal and external areas of the anus, and can also be known as pile or hemorrhoidal lumps. Hemorrhoids are a common and frequently encountered disorder and can be categorized into internal, external and mixed types depending on the location. Internal hemorrhoids are by far the most common. This condition can cause pain around the anus, a sinking and/or distending sensation of the rectum, itching and bleeding.

Point

Erbai (EX-UE 2)

Location

Erbai (EX-UE 2) are two extra points located on the palmar side of each forearm, 4cun proximal to the crease of the wrist and on either sides of the tendon of the radial flexor muscle of the wrist (See Fig. 3-1).

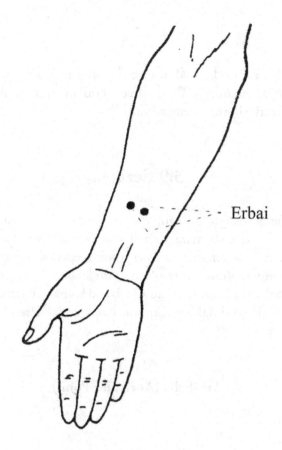

Fig. 3-1 Erbai (EX-UE 2)

Method

Acupuncture is used. Locate Erbai (EX-UE 2) bilaterally, totaling four points. Insert a 1.5cun needle to a depth of 1cun into each point, applying a reducing method for acute cases of hemorrhoid. For chronic cases insert with a reinforcing method, in either case, manipulate the needles until the patient can feel a Qi sensation at local area on the forearm (for about three minutes). Repeat manipulation every five minutes and retain the needles for 30 minutes total. Treat once daily, and one treatment course is equal to two weeks.

Result

99 cases were treated with this method: 64 cases completely resolved and 35 cases slightly improved. Of the 64 cases that completely resolved, 36% improved within one week of treatment and 19% improved within four weeks of treatment.

Case

Tan xx, male 62 year-old, worker: Presented with chronic internal and external hemorrhoids for the past 21 years. He had undergone three operations and frequently presented with bleeding and pain upon defecation. After four weeks of treatment, his symptoms completely resolved with no recurrence for over 10 years.

Discussion

The extra point Erbai (EX-UE 2) is located near to the lung and pericardium meridians, and when needled is close to the Sanjiao meridian. These three meridians can regulate movement of the large intestine, and therefore effectively treat hemorrhoid.

3.9 Eczema

Eczema is a common type of allergic inflammatory dermatitis, and can be divided into acute and chronic presentations. Acute eczema is characterized by a sudden onset of symmetric and polymorphic lesions in a repeated formation, accompanied by erythema, edema, papule, vesiculation, oozing and intense itching. Once the initial phase has resolved, it undergoes decrustation and leaves no trace of irritation. Chronic eczema derives from an acute attack and is characterized by rough skin that is dark red or gray in color, with scales and flaking. Chronic eczema may often bring about acute attacks.

Point

Antihelix (Auricular Point)

Location

Antihelix (auricular point) is located in the center of the antihelix on the ear (See page 203 Auricular point picture).

Method

Cutting therapy is used. First, sterilize the local area of the point with alcohol. With the left hand, stabilize the ear and hold a three-edged needle (or operating scalpel) in the right hand. Make a perpendicular incision horizontally across the antihelix at a length of 0.2-0.4 cm and a depth of 0.1-0.2 cun. Allow the area to bleed 2-3 drops of blood. Apply a cotton plaster for four hours, and then remove. The procedure may be repeated twice weekly.

Result

12 cases were treated with this method: All of the cases completely resolved after 3-4 treatments, with an average treatment length of seven days.

Case

Ding xx, female, 18 years old: Presented with bilateral and contra lateral red papules on the external side of her lower legs, accompanied by vesica, exudation and erosion on an area 8 x 10 cm on the right leg and 6 x 8 cm on the left leg. The borders of the lesions were unclear, with local skin redness and severe pain and itching. Her condition had presented for 15 days. The traditional Chinese medicine diagnosis was eczema from dampness and heat in the spleen and stomach. After five days of treatment by the above method, the local area had returned to normal color and the condition resolved.

Discussion

1. If there is not access to a surgical knife, a three-aged needle may be used.

2. If the patient is against bleeding therapy, a retained needle may be placed on bilateral Antihelix instead. Instruct the patient to press the points 50~100 times, three times per day.

3. For more rapid results, use a three-edged needle to minimally bleed at the local skin lesion.

3.10 Urticaria

Urticaria is a kind of allergic skin disease involving skin wheals as the main manifestation, with a sudden onset and rapid disappearance, often leaving no trace after recovery. During an attack, severe itching and a sensation of burning heat appear on the affected part. Urticaria may repeatedly surface and last for a long time.

Point

Shenque (RN 8)

Location

Shenque (RN 8) is located on the center of the umbilicus.

Method

Cupping therapy is used. Using a large-sized glass cup, place it on umbilicus for three minutes (with vacuum seal). Then, remove it and repeat again after three minutes to complete one treatment. Repeat 2~3 treatments every day.

Result

105 cases were treated with this method. In general, the cases improved after one treatment with a reduction in itching and rash. Complete resolution occurred after 3~4 days of treatment. The total efficacy rate was 96.19%.

Case

Lin xx, male, 45 year-old, officer: Presented with itching and a rash all over his body, particularly on his back. He was diagnosed with urticaria from wind and heat. He was treated with the above method. The itching and rash decreased after two treatments and the condition completely resolved after one more subsequent treatment.

Discussion

Urticaria is usually a result of suppressed immune function. Stimulation of the point Shenque (RN 8) can increase immune function in the body.

3.11 Cutaneous Pruritus

Cutaneous pruritus is a kind of dermatitis, which has a sensation of itching on the affected part but with no primary skin lesion. It is caused by a functional disorder of the cutaneous sensory nerve. Clinical manifestations include severe paroxysmal itching of the skin, which is usually worse at night or a result of irritating food or emotional upset. During an attack, the itching is often very difficult to bear or alleviate. Once the itching has ceased, there is no remaining evidence of attack.

Point

Xuehai (SP 10)

Location

Xuehai (SP 10) is located when the knee is flexed. The point is 2cun above the medial-superior border of the patella, on the bulge of the medial portion of the quadriceps femoris muscle. The point may also be located by cupping your right palm over the left knee when the patient's knee is flexed, with the thumb placed on the medial side of the leg and the other four fingers directed upwards. The thumb should form an angle of 45° with the index finger, and the point lies where the tip of the thumb rests.

Method

Acupuncture is used. Locate the points bilaterally. Insert 1.5cun needles to a depth of 1cun at each point. Apply a reducing method for excess patterns and a reinforcing method for deficient patterns.

Retain the needles for 30 minutes, and repeat once daily. One course of treatment is equal to 10 sessions. Improved results typically appear after three courses of treatment.

Result

30 cases were treated with this method for 4–30 treatments: 19 cases completely resolved; nine cases slightly improved; and two cases had no effect. The total efficacy rate was 93.3%.

Case

Zhu xx, female, 54 year-old Officer: Presented with itching over her entire body for one year, upon examination, papule and scratch marks could be found on her abdomen and arms. Her symptoms were limited to severe itching, with no systemic disorder. She was diagnosed with cutaneous pruritis. After five treatments with the above method, the itching had subsided. After fifteen treatments, the condition had completely resolved.

3.12 Psoriasis

Psoriasis is a type of chronic erythroderma desquamativum. Clinical manifestations include red, scaly lesions combined with severe itching. Psoriasis is considered a chronic condition and can therefore recur. It most commonly affects young or middle-aged people.

Point

Ear Apex (EP-K 12)

Location

Ear Apex (EP-K 12) is an auricular point located at the upper tip of the auricle and superior to the helix when the ear is folded towards the tragus (See page 203 Auricular point picture).

Method

Acupuncture is used. First, use a three-edged needle to prick and bleed the point. Then, insert a 1cun needle horizontally and toward the helix to a depth of 0.5–0.8cun. Lift and rotate the needle several times over the course of 30 minutes. Repeat the treatment once daily or every other day, until the symptoms have resolved.

Result

50 cases were treated with this method: 32 cases completely resolved; 16 cases slightly improved; and two cases showed no effect.

Case

Zhang xx, male, 15 year-old student: Presented with a few red, small papules on his forehead with itching that began three months prior. After 2~3 days from the initial onset, silvery white scales began to sluff off, the itching continued and the lesions spread to cover 30% of his body. He was diagnosed with psoriasis. He was treated with the above method for ten treatments, after which the scales began to disappear. Treatment continued for five more treatments, and all of the papules disappeared with marked improvement.

3.13 Acne

Acne is a chronic inflammation of the hair follicles and sebaceous glands on the skin. It often occurs among boys and girls during adolescence, and may be referred to as adolescent acne. Clinical manifestations include red papules or nodules, which occur most often on the face.

Point

Dazhui (DU 14)

Location

Dazhui (DU 14) is located below the spinous process of the seventh cervical vertebra, approximately at the level of the top of the shoulders.

Method

Three-edged needle and cupping therapy are used. Have the patient seated with arms outstretched onto a table. Tap a three-edged needle for 1~2 pricks and at a depth of 2~3mm. Gently squeeze the point to let some blood out, and then apply a cup for 15 minutes (a total of 2~3 ml of blood should collect). Remove the cup and repeat the entire treatment every other day. One course equals four treatments.

Result

39 cases were treated with this method: 29 cases completely resolved; seven cases slightly improved; and three cases had no effect.

Case

Zhang xx, female, 20 year-old student: Presented with acne for the past four years, with many red papules on her face, particularly on her forehead. She had taken various medications, with no result. She was diagnosed with acne. After one treatment, no new lesions had appeared. After ten more treatments, all the papules had disappeared, but her face had a deep color on the skin. After three months, the skin had cleared completely.

3.14 Vitiligo

Vitiligo is an acquired skin disease resulting in localized pigment loss, which is characterized by irregular white patches on the skin and without subjective uncomfortable symptom.

Point

Local area

Location

Local area refers to the center of the affected area.

Method

Moxibustion is used. Cut a piece of paper with a small hole in the center and place it on the skin with the affected area appearing in the center. Apply a moxa stick to the local area until it becomes red in color, and the patient cannot bear the heat any more. After 30 treatments, improvement is often visible. This disorder usually occurs on various places on the body. Treatment may be applied on one specific area at a time, and then one by one until normal skin color is restored.

Result

Six cases were treated with this method, all of which completely resolved. The average success rate occurred within 25~38 treatments.

Cases

Li xx, male, 42 year-old, officer: Presented with two white patches (3cm in diameter) on the left side of his forehead for the past three years. He was diagnosed with vitiligo. After treatment with the above method for 28 sessions, the condition resolved.

Chapter IV Obstetrical, Gynecological and Pediatric Diseases

4.1 Dysfunctional Uterine Bleeding

Dysfunctional uterine bleeding is a common gynecological disease, and may result in abnormal uterine bleeding caused by ovarian dysfunction. Clinical manifestations include abnormalities of the menstrual cycle, including prolonged and/or heavy bleeding.

Point

Duanhong (Experiential Point)

Location

Duanhong (experiential point) is located between the knuckles of the second and third fingers (See Fig. 4-1).

Method

Acupuncture and moxibustion are used. Apply both acupuncture and moxibustion to the point Duanhong (experiential point) bilaterally, after sterilizing with 75% alcohol. Insert 1.5 ~ 2cun needles horizontally to a depth of 1~2cun into each point. Manipulate with a reinforcing method. Once the patient can feel a Qi sensation as a slight surging of energy, stop manipulating the needle and let it remain untouched for the next twenty minutes. During this time, apply a moxa stick in a circular motion around the point for 10~15 minutes. Repeat this treatment once a day. Ten treatments make up one course.

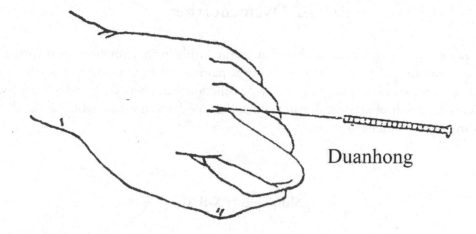

Fig. 4-1 Duanhong (Experiential Point)

Result

Usually one course of this treatment will regulate the menstrual cycle. If the patient has not improved after the first course of treatment, pause for three days, and then begin a second course.

Case

Wang xx, female, 33 years of age: Presented with continual bleeding for more than one month. The quality of the menstruate was thin, the amount was sometimes profuse and sometimes scanty and the color was pale. She used western medicine in an attempt to stop the bleeding for 13 days, with no effect. She began to feel dizzy, weak, chronic fatigue, lassitude, a sallow complexion and pale lips. Her traditional Chinese medicine diagnosis was dysfunctional uterine bleeding as a result of spleen deficiency. One hour after the above treatment, her bleeding has decreased. After the second treatment, the patient experienced no further dysfunctional uterine bleeding. Nevertheless, one complete course was recommended to reinforce the treatment, in an effort to prevent recurrence.

Discussion

This method is suitable to treat dysfunctional uterine bleeding due to spleen deficiency. For optimum results, the patient should feel a warm (Qi) sensation travel from the knuckles to the elbow, or even the shoulder. The point Duanhong has the special function of stopping bleeding, especially in the uterus, and links to all meridians. When the circulation of Qi is good, it can control the blood so the blood stays within the vessels.

4.2 Dysmenorrhea

Dysmenorrhea refers to periodic lower abdominal pain during, prior to or after the menstrual period. In severe cases, fainting may ensue as a result of the pain. It has been customary to classify cases of dysmenorrhea into two main groups: primary or functional dysmenorrhea, which is of unknown etiology and not a result of another disease; and secondary dysmenorrhea, which is the direct result of disorder in the reproductive system.

Point

Shiqizhui (EX-B 8)

Location

Shiqizhui (EX-B 8) is an extra point is located below the spinous process of the fifth lumbar vertebra (See Fig. 4-2).

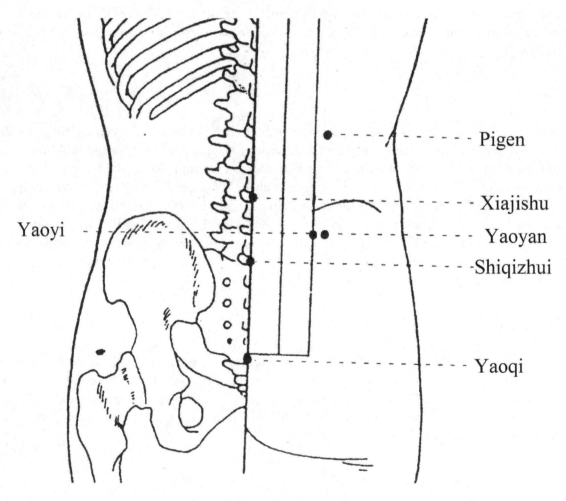

Fig. 4-2 Shiqizhui (EX-B 8)

Method

Acupuncture and moxibustion are used. Have the patient lie in a prone position. Locate the point, swab with alcohol, and insert a 2-2.5 cun needle perpendicularly about 2 cun. Once the patient can feel a Qi sensation around the local area, quickly rotate the needle to strongly stimulate until the sensation travels to the lower abdomen. Continue manipulating the needle for 1-2 minutes, until the pain decreases and stops. Retain the needle for 20 minutes without manipulation. If the patient's symptoms do not improve, warm the needle with moxibustion and leave the needle retained for 10 more minutes.

Results

64 cases were treated with this method: 59 cases completely resolved; four cases achieved very good results; and one case had no effect.

Case

Liu xx, female, 17 year-old student: Presented with severe, twisting pain in her lower abdomen with her menstruation since her first cycle came at 17 years old. Other symptoms included nausea, vomiting, and soreness of the low back. Her abdominal pain continued for two hours during her menstruation. The TCM diagnosis for this patient was dysmenorrhea due to stagnation of Qi and blood. After one treatment with the above method, her pain decreased within one minute. After three minutes, the pain had ceased.

Discussion

This point, Shiqizhui (EX-B 8), is located in the lumbar region, along the Du meridian. The Du meridian controls all the yang of the body, and is known as the sea of the Yang meridians. Shiqizhui (EX-B 8) has the function to regulate all the Yang Qi within all the Yang meridians, to alleviate stagnation and reduce pain. From a western viewpoint, this point directly relates to the nervous system connecting with the uterine muscle. Pressing on the point can stimulate the nervous system, relaxing the muscles and alleviating spasms felt from muscle contraction.

4.3 Leukorrhagia

Leukorrhagia is a disorder characterized by persistent and excessive vaginal discharge (also known as leukorrhea). The discharge may have an abnormal color, quality and smell; and may also be accompanied by other constitutional or local symptoms.

Point

Sihua (Experiential Point)

Location

Sihua (experiential point) is located on the back, and consists of four points. The four points make the shape of a flower, located 1.5 cun on either side of the spinal column, just below T7 and T10 (See Fig. 4-3).

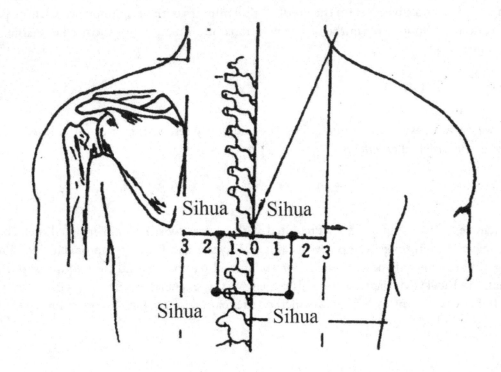

Fig. 4-3 Sihua (Experiential Point)

Method

Acupuncture is used with the patient lying in a prone position. Insert a 1.5 cun needle obliquely into each point, angled toward the mid-line and at a depth of about 1.0 cun. If the leukorrhea is yellow or red, apply a reducing method. If the leukorrhea is clear or white and accompanied by dizziness, palpitation or low back pain, apply a reinforcing method. When the patient can feel a Qi sensation, stop manipulation and retain the needles for 20 minutes. A patient with a deficiency syndrome may need 40 minutes or more with the needles to appropriately tonify (the length of retention will ultimately depend on individual constitution). Repeat the treatment once a day. The treatment can be performed whether or not the patient is menstruating.

Result

28 cases were treated with this method for 1-6 treatments, with an average of three treatments. Of the 28 cases, 20 complained of white leukorrhea, six reported yellow leukorrhea, and two cases had red leukorrhea: 21 cases completely resolved; six cases slightly improved; and one case had no change.

Case

Yuan xx, female, 25 years of age: Presented with leukorrhagia for the past six months, feelings of dizziness, palpitation, hunger, fatigue, and weakness. The traditional Chinese medicine diagnosis was leukorrhagia due to spleen Qi deficiency. After three treatments with the above method, the discharge had ceased. After another week without treatment, the patient's remaining symptoms disappeared.

4.4 Infertility

Primary infertility is when a couple is unable to conceive a child after two years of attempt through unprotected intercourse. Secondary infertility is an inability for a couple to conceive a second time, two years after a previous childbirth, miscarriage or abortion.

Point

Guanyuan (RN 4)

Location

Guanyuan (RN 4) is located on the anterior midline, 3 cun below the umbilicus.

Method

Indirect moxibustion with ginger is used. Slice a piece of fresh ginger about 2 cm in diameter and 2-3mm in thickness. Make holes within the ginger slice and place it over the point Guanyuan (RN 4). Then, place a large cone of moxa on top of the ginger. Ignite and allow the cone to burn fully and replace with a fresh cone, for a total of five cones. Repeat the entire treatment twice daily, once in the morning and once in the evening. Ten treatments are equal to one course. Usually, only one to five treatment courses are necessary. During a women's menstruation, abstain from this treatment.

Result

30 cases of primary infertility were treated with this method for five courses of treatment: 11 women conceived a child within a year.

Case

Wang xx, female, age 24: Presented with an inability to conceive a child after four years of trying with her husband. She noted feeling constantly depressed, cold, fatigued and with no appetite. Her Western medical doctor diagnosed her with twisted fallopian tubes and suggested an operation, which she did not want to have. Therefore, she sought Traditional Chinese Medicine treatment, which diagnosed her with kidney Qi and Yang deficiency. After five courses of the moxibustion treatment described above, she became pregnant. Eight months later, she had a baby.

Discussion

The point Guanyuan (RN 4) is located on the Ren meridian, which has a relationship with the Du and Chong Meridians as all three intersect at Guanyuan (RN 4). Applying moxa on this point can warm and stimulate all of them. The Chong, Du and Ren Meridians are responsible for physiological gynecological function.

4.5 Pelvic Inflammatory Disease

Pelvic Inflammatory Disease (PID) is a chronic or acute inflammation of the internal female reproductive organs (uterus, fallopian tubes and ovaries), the connective tissue of the region and the peritoneum. According to traditional Chinese medicine, PID falls into the categories of *Re Ru Xueshi* (Heat Invading the Blood Chamber/Uterus), *Dai Xiai* (Leukorrhagia), and *Zheng Jiai* (Abdominal Mass).

Point

Guilai (ST 29)

Location

Guilai (ST 29) is located 4cun below the umbilicus, 2cun lateral to Zhongji (RN 3).

Method

Acupressure therapy is used. Have the patient lie in a relaxed supine position, with knees bent and feet flat on the table or floor. Apply pressure onto bilateral Guilai (ST 29), with an outward-circular rotation for a hundred repetitions. Then, press and rotate in an inward-circular motion on the points for another hundred repetitions. Finally, directly press on Guilai (ST 29) for fifty repetitions. This treatment should be self-administered by the patient once a day, before going to bed.

Result

37 cases were treated with the above method. Of that, the average length of chronic pelvic inflammation was four years, with treatment frequency ranging between 9 ~ 46 times (at an average rate of 25.03 treatments): 20 cases completely resolved; 12 cases had improved; and five cases had no change.

Case

Zhang xx, female, 43 year-old worker: Presented with lower abdominal and lower back pain, as well as foul-smelling red leukorrhea for the past three years. All of these symptoms had significantly worsened in the past week, which prompted her to seek treatment. Of late, it was difficult for her to walk and the pain worsened with abdominal pressure. The traditional Chinese medicine diagnosis was chronic pelvic inflammation due to stagnation of Qi and blood. After applying the above acupressure cycle for 22 treatments, her pain was gone. Physical examination showed that her condition had alleviated, and by her annual follow-up had not recurred since.

Discussion

The point Guilai (ST 29) is on the Yangming (Stomach) Meridian. The Yangming Meridian channels are more full of blood and Qi than any other meridian in the body. In addition, Guilai (ST 29) is located on the lower abdomen, and is therefore even more effective. By applying acupressure on this point, the circulation of Qi and blood in the pelvic floor is invigorated and will help to remove any stagnation. Where there is stagnation, there is pain; and when the stagnation is gone, so is the pain.

4.6 Morning sickness

Morning sickness is marked by a group of symptoms including nausea, vomiting, dizziness and anorexia within the first trimester of gestation. It is most commonly seen during the early stage of pregnancy, and contrary to the title, symptoms can occur at anytime of day. Severe morning sickness may emaciate and dehydrate the pregnant woman very quickly, triggering other complications and/or requiring hospitalization.

Point

Shenmen (EP-I 1)

Location

Shenmen (EP-I 1) is an auricular point located at the bifurcating area between the superior and inferior antihelix crus, and at the lateral 1/3 of triangular fossa (See page 203 Auricular Point Picture).

Method

Auricular acupuncture is used. Insert small, 3mm dermal needles into bilateral Shenmen (EP-I 1). Cover the needles with a five mm square plaster, replacing the needles every five days. Stop treatment once the condition has resolved, usually within two weeks (five treatments). Instruct the patient to press the needles with their fingers 50 times on each point in the morning, afternoon and evening. If nausea or discomfort arises throughout the day, the needles may be pressed during that time to ease the discomfort.

Result

124 cases were treated with the above method: 64 cases completely resolved within one treatment; 39 cases completely resolved within two treatments; and 21 cases completely resolved within three treatments.

Discussion

Shenmen (auricular point EP-I 1) can stimulate the auricular branch of the Vagus nerve, therefore regulating digestive muscles.

4.7 Abnormal Position of the Fetus

This condition arises when the fetus is abnormally positioned for labor within the uterus after thirty weeks of pregnancy. It is often seen in multipara or pregnant women who have laxity of the abdominal wall. There are no subjective symptoms as far as the pregnant woman is concerned with an abnormally positioned fetus, and precise diagnosis is confirmed by ultrasound and/or obstetric examination. Possible abnormal presentations include breech position or transverse position.

Point

Zhiyin (BL 67)

Location

Zhiyin (BL 67) is located on the lateral side of the small toe, about 0.1cun from the corner of the nail.

Method

Moxibustion is used. Have the patient in a relaxed, seated position; with her pant-waist loosened and feet elevated onto a stool. Ignite a moxa stick, and apply over the points bilaterally. Use a sparrow pecking for 20 minutes on each side, once or twice a day. Seven days of treatment is one course.

Result

100 cases were treated with this method: 71 cases were successful and 29 cases had no result. In most of the successful cases, the fetus had turned within three days: 24 cases succeeded on the first day of treatment; 17 cases on the second day; 13 cases on the third day; nine cases after four or five days; five cases after six or seven days of treatment; and three cases after eight to nine days.

Case

Li xx, female, 23 years of age: Presented with a horizontal fetal position in her seventh month of pregnancy with her first child. Her obstetrician discovered that her abdominal wall was very tight and the amniotic fluid levels were within normal limits. Her traditional Chinese medicine diagnosis was abnormal positioning of the fetus due to imbalance of the Chong and Ren Meridians. The above moxibustion protocol was used, with the patient continuing self-treatment at home once a day. After three days, the fetal position had changed back to normal (head-down), and the baby was born during the 38th week.

Discussion

Mal-positioned fetus has a close relationship with Kidney Qi, which thus controls the blood (a major foundation for women). When Qi and blood are balanced, the position of the baby will be normal. Fetal growth depends on the Chong, Ren, and Dai meridians, and these three meridians also have a close relationship with the kidney. The urinary bladder relates very closely to the kidney, as an internal/external pair. Zhiyin (BL 67) point is on the urinary bladder meridian and has the function to regulate kidney Qi, thus harmonizing the Chong, Ren and Dai meridians. Once in balance again, the fetal position will also normalize.

4.8 Prolonged or Difficult Labor

Prolonged or difficult labor refers to a hypodynamic contraction of the uterus once labor as begun. Clinical manifestations include a short duration of uterine contractions, irregular intervals between contractions, and a non-progressive cervical dilation and/or fetal station (inability of the fetus to move progressively down the birth canal). All of the above will lead to a prolonged and difficult labor.

Point

Hegu (LI 4)

Location

Hegu (LI 4) is located on the dorsum of the hand, between the 1st and 2nd metacarpal bones and approximately in line with the midpoint of the 2nd metacarpal bone on the radial side.

Method

Electrical stimulation acupuncture is used. Have the laboring woman lie in a supine position with both legs up. Insert a 1.5 cun needle into bilateral Hegu (LI 4), perpendicularly and to a depth of 1.2 cun. Angle the needle toward the point Huoxi (SI 3). Once the patient can feel a heavy Qi sensation, apply an e-stimulation machine electrode to the needle with a continuous wave pattern. Continue this treatment until the baby is born.

Result

30 cases were treated with this method: within 5~10 minutes, contractions and cervical dilation began to progress in all cases, thus promoting a smoother childbirth.

Case

Zhao xx, female, 43 years old and pregnant with her fourth child: Presented with difficult labor as a result of stunted cervical dilation. After treatment with the above method for 30 minutes, her contractions became more intense, consistent, and the baby was born shortly thereafter.

Discussion

The point Hegu (LI 4) belongs to Yangming (large intestine) meridian, and specifically, is the Yuan-Source point for this meridian. It can treat difficult labor by strengthening the uterine muscle, and must only be used in pregnant women during labor.

4.9 Postpartum Retention of Urine

Postpartum retention of urine most often is the result of a difficult labor, which has lead to loss of nerve function in the reproductive area - giving rise to large amounts of urine being retained in the bladder. Clinically, it is characterized by distension and fullness in the lower abdomen due to blocked urinary flow.

Point

Shenque (RN 8)

Location

Shenque (RN 8) is located in the center of the umbilicus.

Method

Indirect moxibustion with salt is used. Have the patient lie in a supine position. Dry-fry 20g of salt until it turns a yellow color and place it into the navel, completely covering the umbilicus (forming a circle on the abdomen about 2-3 cm in diameter). Then, grind two chopped green onions into a paste and form into a cake 0.3 mm high and place it on top of the salt. Finally, place a large moxa cone on top of the green onion cake. Ignite the moxa cone and allow it to burn slightly more than half way. Repeat with the other cones until the patient has a desire to urinate, or the area becomes too hot for the patient to tolerate. Usually, three to five moxa cones will be sufficient, and there is no need to repeat once urinary flow has resumed.

Result

19 cases were treated with this method: 10 cases completely resolved after one moxa cone was burned; five cases resolved after three or four moxa cones were burned; one case resolved within four hours

post-treatment; one case resolved after two treatments on consecutive days; and two cases underwent three treatments with no improvement.

Case

Luo xx, female, 25 years of age: Presented with no desire to urinate for two days after the birth of her child. First, she was treated by Western medications with no result, then, the doctor would drain her bladder every four hours via a urinary catheter. After one treatment with three moxa cones, she felt the need to urinate. By the second day of treatment, when two moxa cones were used, she was able to urinate normally.

4.10 Postpartum Complications

After childbirth, it is possible for the mother to experience complications such as nervousness, anger, excessive worry, fatigue and weakness. All of these symptoms are often the result of blood loss, and lead to insomnia.

Point

Baihui (DU 20)

Location

Baihui (DU 20) is located on the head, 5 cun directly above the midpoint of the anterior hairline, approximately on the midpoint of the line connecting the apexes of both ears.

Method

Moxibustion is used. With the patient in a seated position, spread the hair on top of the head to expose the point. Ignite a moxa stick and hold it above the point, using sparrow-pecking and circular techniques. This treatment is best when applied 15 minutes before going to sleep. Four treatments are equal to one course. Repeat as long as necessary.

Result

21 cases were treated with this method: most of the patients were able to sleep after 15 minutes of treatment; a few patients could sleep within a few hours after treatment; and some patients fell asleep during the treatment. In general, all cases were able to sleep soundly for 8~12 hours.

Case

Luo xx, female 23 years old: Presented with difficulty sleeping for the past two days, since the birth of her child (which was a difficult labor and resulted in a lot of blood loss). She took barbiturates as prescribed by her Western doctor, with no effect. The first time she was treated with the above method, she fell asleep for six hours within two hours after treatment. After the second treatment, she fell asleep for eight hours after thirty minutes of treatment. By the third treatment, she fell asleep during the treatment, and stayed asleep for nine more hours.

Discussion

Baihui (DU 20) belongs to the Du meridian. The Du meridian controls all of the Yang meridians of the body. After labor, a woman tends to be Qi and blood deficient, because of the immense expenditure of energy and loss of blood. Baihui (DU 20) can increase Yang and Qi to quiet the mother's mind and promote restful sleep.

4.11 Hypogalactia (Insufficient Lactation)

Hypogalactia happens when very little or no milk is able to secrete from the breast of a nursing mother. Clinical manifestations include scanty flow or absence of milk secretion after childbirth, or a continuous decrease in milk quantity during lactation. It is commonly known as "Insufficient Lactation."

Point

Danzhong (Shanzhong) (RN 17)

Location

Danzhong (RN 17) is located on the anterior midline, at the level with the 4th inter-costal space, midway between the nipples.

Method

Acupuncture and moxibustion are used. Have the patient lie in a supine position. Insert a 2 cun needle horizontally and angled down towards the feet, to a depth of 1.5 cun. Once the patient can feel a Qi sensation, leave the needle untouched for 30~60 minutes (depending on the severity of the case). If due to cold or excess pathology, retain the needle for a longer time. If due to deficiency or heat, retain the needle for a shorter duration. For both deficient and cold syndromes, apply moxibustion using a sparrow-pecking method for 20 minutes after the needle is removed.

Result

20 cases were treated with the above method, all with successful results: 14 cases produced sufficient milk after the first treatment; five cases produced sufficient milk after the second treatment; and one case produced sufficient milk after the third treatment.

Case

Gui xx, female, 24 years of age: Presented with breast distension and pain, difficulty excreting milk, and heightened anxiety and depression after the birth of her child. Her tongue was red with a yellow coat and her pulse was wiry. Her traditional Chinese medicine diagnosis was insufficient lactation as a result of stagnation of liver Qi. After two treatments with the above method, her milk flowed smoothly to nourish the baby.

Discussion

Danzhong (RN 17) is one of eight connecting points, and is also the commander of Qi for the entire body. Qi can regulate milk flow in nursing mothers and stimulate endocrine function. If there is Qi deficiency or stagnation, this point can either cause an increase or decrease in milk flow. By stimulating Danzhong (RN 17), Qi circulation is regulated so milk can flow smoothly.

4.12 Childhood Mumps

Childhood mumps (epidemic parotitis or mumps) is an acute infectious disease, defined as an acute, general and non-suppurative disease caused by the mumps virus. Characteristics include swelling and pain of the parotid gland.

Point

Jiaosun (SJ 20)

Location

Jiaosun (SJ 20) is located directly above the ear apex, within the hairline.

Methods

1. Acupressure is used. Using the thumb and index finger, pinch and apply pressure to the points bilaterally and from both directions, for about 50 repetitions. Apply pressure as much as the child can tolerate. Repeat this treatment once daily and three treatments constitute one course.

2. Burning therapy is used. Place a small piece of cotton, soaked in cooking oil, on the bottom end of a match. Clean the local area and cut any hair around the point. Ignite the cotton, once the flame has gone out touch the cotton to the skin at Jiaosun (SJ 20). As soon as you hear a sound from the child, quickly remove the cotton from the point. The burnt area should be marked by a 0.5 cm square. After a few days, a scar will develop. Keep the local area dry and clean, it will heal on its own.

3. Bleeding therapy is used. Insert a three-edged needle into the point on the affected side for one to three quick pricks (at a depth of 0.2~0.5 cm). A small amount of blood should release.

Apply dry cotton to close the hole and clean up the blood. One treatment is usually sufficient, but if after two days there is no improvement, repeat the treatment.

Results

Method 1. 12 cases were treated with the first method and after one course, all cases completely resolved.

Method 2. 334 cases were treated with the second method: 312 cases completely resolved; five cases improved; and 17 cases showed no effect.

Method 3. Usually one treatment will resolve all symptoms, but two or three treatments may be used if necessary.

Cases

1. Guo xx, male, six years old: Presented with mumps on the left side of his neck, distension and swelling below the affected ear and an inability to open his mouth easily. The skin color around the area was normal in color and his pain increased with pressure. The traditional Chinese medicine diagnosis was childhood mumps due to wind heat. After three treatments with the first method, his symptoms had completely resolved.

2. Wang xx, male, four years old: Presented with mumps on both sides of his neck, which pressed on the tendons causing so much pain that he could not eat. The traditional Chinese medicine diagnosis was childhood mumps due to wind heat. After 30 minutes of treatment on both sides with the second method, he could eat fruit and drink water. By the next day, and after no further treatment, his symptoms had completely resolved.

3. Chen xx, male, five years old: Presented with mumps on the right side of his neck for two days, which were swollen and felt warm and painful when touched. In addition, he had a fever, headache, and difficulty opening his mouth. The traditional Chinese medicine diagnosis was childhood mumps due to wind heat. After one treatment with the third method, the pain and fever were gone. The mumps had completely resolved after three treatments.

Discussion

Method one is appropriate for mild cases; methods two and three are more appropriate for severe cases; and method two will only need to be done once.

4.13 Infantile Diarrhea

Infantile diarrhea refers to a sudden increase in frequency and volume of defecation in infants, and may be associated with improper food intake, or a bacterial or viral infection. Chronic presentations usually occur over the course of four weeks and are often the result of uncontrolled intestinal infections or intestinal flora imbalance resulting from overused antibiotics.

Point

Shenque (RN 8)

Location

Shenque (RN 8) is located in the center of the umbilicus.

Method

Medicated compress therapy is used. Make an herbal formula of equal amounts of the following ground herbs: Gan Jiang (Dried Ginger, *Rhizoma Zingieris*); Fu Zi (Prepared Lateral Root of Aconite, *Radix Aconiti Lateralis Prasparata*); and Wu Zhu Yu, (Evodia Fruit, *Fructus Euodiae*). Combine the powdered herbs into a thick paste with vinegar. Fill the navel with the paste and cover the umbilicus with a 4cm square plaster. Change it after three days and be careful keep the area dry while the plaster is in place.

Result

32 cases were treated with the above method: 31 cases completely resolved and one case did not change. Of the 31 successful cases: 21 cases resolved after two days of treatment; eight cases resolved after three days of treatment; and two cases resolved after five days of treatment.

Case

Ai xx, female, six months old: Presented with 7-9 bouts of diarrhea per day, for the past 15 days. The stool contained undigested food and the girl was thin, with a sallow complexion and a poor appetite. Her tongue was light red with a slightly thick, sticky white coating. Her traditional Chinese medicine diagnosis was diarrhea due to deficient Qi and spleen yang. By the second day of this treatment, the child's diarrhea had reduced to three or four times in a day. By the third day, normal bowel movements had resumed.

Discussion

Shenque (RN 8) belongs to the Ren meridian and has a special function to strengthen the spleen and stomach. Fu Zi and Wu Zhu Yu improve Yang while Gan Jiang removes cold from the meridians. Improving Yang and removing cold together have the result of stopping diarrhea.

4.14 Enuresis

Childhood enuresis is defined as an involuntary emptying of the bladder during the daytime or at night, in children above the age of three. Nocturnal enuresis is usually accompanied by vivid dreams - either several times in a night or once every few nights. In chronic cases, there are accompanying symptoms of sallow complexion, anorexia and lassitude. This disease is categorized as "Yi Niao" (bed-wetting) in traditional Chinese medicine.

Point

Yiniao (Experiential Point)

Location

Yiniao (experiential point) is located in the middle of the most distal crease of the small toe (See Fig. 4-4).

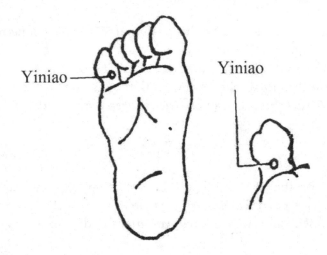

Fig. 4-4 Yiniao (Experiential Point)

Method

Acupuncture is used. Sterilize the points bilaterally with 75% alcohol. While rotating, insert 0.5cun needles until the tip of the needle touches the bone. Then, manually manipulate the needles strongly, by rotating until the patient feels severe pain in the local area, with heat and distension sensations traveling to the lower abdomen. Leave the needles untouched for 30 minutes. Treatment should be done once daily. Five treatments constitute one course.

Result

10 cases were treated with this method: five cases completely resolved after one treatment; three cases completely resolved after two treatments; and two cases completely resolved after three treatments.

Case

Zhao xx, female, 15 years old: Presented with enuresis every day or every other day, for the past 10 years. She was treated by many methods, without any result. When she was given acupuncture, she improved after one treatment. The same night that she was treated, she did not involuntarily urinate (even after ingesting watermelon). After two courses of treatment, the enuresis had completely resolved and had not returned by her follow-up seven years later.

Discussion

The most important thing in this treatment is patient cooperation. During the treatment, children are advised to limit their activity and avoid drinking liquids or eating watery fruits before bed. In addition, regular (fixed) bed times, and toilet schedules are important, especially at night.

4.15 Excessive Night Crying

This condition presents as interval or continuous crying throughout the night, while the child maintains a pleasant disposition throughout the day. It may be caused by abdominal pain, abdominal distension, anal itching/discomfort, over-eating, indigestion or a nervous system disorder - all of which can lead to excessive crying at night.

Point

Zhongchong (PC 9)

Location

Zongchong (PC 9) is located in the center of the tip of the middle finger.

Method

Bleeding therapy is used. Sterilize the area of Zhongchong (PC 9) on one side. Then, insert a three-edge needle to a depth of 0.1cun. Allow for four drops of blood to be released. Usually one treatment will yield a good result, but if the treatment is not successful, the treatment may be performed on the opposite side the following day. Two treatments should be enough to solve the problem.

Result

49 cases were treated with this method: 46 cases completely resolved; and three cases found no change.

Case

Zhou xx, female, three years old: Presented with unceasing crying all night long and normal disposition during the daytime. After she was treated once by the above method, she slept through the night without any crying.

Chapter V: Ophthalmic, Ear-Nose-Throat Diseases and Others

5.1 Hordeolum

Hordeolum, or a common stye, is a kind of suppurative inflammation of the eyelid. After suppuration, the pustule head is a whitish-yellow color and in the shape of a ripe wheat-seed (in Chinese, "mai li zhong"). If tarsadenitis occurs after suppuration, a pus head can be seen on the surface of the palpebral conjunctiva, which is known as an internal hordeolum (or, "nei mai li zhong").

Point

Ear Apex (EP-K 12)

Location

Ear apex (EP-K 12) is an auricular point located at the upper tip of the auricle and just superior to the helix when the ear is folded towards the tragus (See page 203 Auricular Point Picture).

Method

Bleeding therapy with a three-edged needle is used. On the affected side, quickly insert a three-edged needle into auricular apex (EP-K 12) to a depth of 0.1cun. Apply pressure to allow between 10-15 drops of blood to produce. When finished, cover the area with dry cotton. Usually one treatment is enough, but the treatment may be repeated two or three more times if needed.

Result

102 cases were treated with this method: 91 cases resolved within one treatment; five cases resolved after two treatments; and six cases were unchanged.

Case

Chen xx, female, 10 years old: Presented with a small knot the size of a grain of rice on the outer edge of her left upper eye. The eye was red, swollen, distended, and painful around the affected area. The traditional Chinese medicine diagnosis was hordeolum due to heat in the stomach meridian. All of her symptoms had resolved by the next day after one treatment with the above method.

Discussion

This disease usually results from heat in the Yangming meridian. All yang meridians connect on the ear, so this point can clear heat from all Yang meridians.

5.2 Lacrimation (Tearing)

Lacrimation refers to excessive tearing due to hyperactive function of the lacrimal glands (tear ducts). A constant running of tears may occur when exposed to wind, and not necessarily include redness or pain of the eyes. Lacrimation is fairly common, most often affecting the elderly. Other conditions that lacrimation may accompany include: dystopy of the lacumal punctum, canaliculitis, trachoma and chronic conjunctivitis.

Point

Taiyang (EX-HN 5)

Location

Taiyang (EX-HN 5) is an extra point located in the depression about one fingerbreadth posterior to the midpoint between the lateral end of the eyebrow and the outer canthus (See Fig. 5-1).

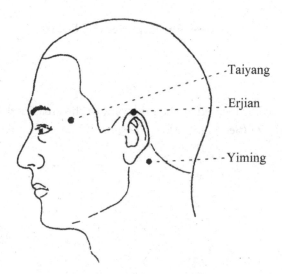

Fig. 5-1 Taiyang (EX-HN 5)

Method

Acupuncture and cupping are used. Perpendicularly insert a 1.0 cun needle into Taiyang (EX-HN 5) on the affected side, at a depth of 0.8 cun. Once the patient can feel a Qi sensation around the eye, leave the needle for 20-30 minutes. After removing the needle, apply gentle cupping on the area for about 15 minutes, using small cups.

Result

27 cases (51 eyes) were treated with the above method (some cases had the problem in only one eye, and others had problems with both eyes simultaneously): 22 cases (41 problem eyes) completely resolved after one treatment; three cases (six problem eyes) slightly improved after one treatment; and the remaining two cases (four problem eyes) did not respond.

Case

Yang xx, male, 38 years old: Presented with continuous lacrimation for the past two years, affecting both eyes and worsening in the winter. The condition made him hesitant to go outside or ride a bicycle. Treatment by western medicine had no effect. After being treated once by this combined acupuncture and cupping method, his symptoms resolved.

5.3 Optic Atrophy

Optic atrophy is a chronic eye disorder marked by gradual degeneration of visual acuity. At the early stage blurring of vision is the only symptom, but at later stages the eyesight may be totally lost.

Point

Xinming (Experiential Point)

Location

Xinming (experiential point) is located at the midpoint of the crease behind the ear, 0.5cun superior and anterior to Yifeng (SJ 17) (See Fig. 5-2).

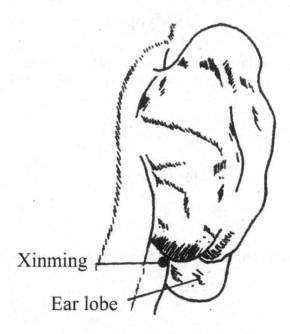

Fig. 5-2 Xinming (Experiential Point)

Method

Acupuncture is used. Fold the patient's ear forward and insert 1.5 cun needles at an oblique angle of 45° along the posterior crease, to a depth of 1cun. Manipulate with a reinforcing method by lifting and thrusting until a Qi sensation can be felt around the eye. Retain the needles without further manipulation for 30 minutes.

Result

698 cases (1252 problem eyes) were treated with the above method: 103 eyes completely resolved; 112 eyes significantly improved; 586 eyes slightly improved; 451 eyes were unchanged. The total efficacy rate was 63.98%.

Case

Yang xx, female, 10 year-old student: Presented with unclear vision in her right eye for the past six years. Western medicine diagnosed her with optic atrophy of the right eye. Her traditional Chinese medicine diagnosis was deficiency of Qi and blood, after treatment with the above method for 100 sessions, her clarity of vision increased and her scope of vision widened (where she had previously only had tunnel vision).

5.4 Myopia

Myopia is an ophthalmology condition mainly characterized by the ability to see near or close objects, but not distant ones. There is no abnormality visible on the outer eyes, and such a condition often affects young people.

Point

Eye (EP-A 10)

Location

Eye (EP-A 10) is an auricular point located in the 5th section of the ear lobe (See page 203 Auricular Point Picture).

Method

Auricular acupuncture is used. Place small press needles (3mm in size) bilaterally into the points and cover them with a 5 mm square plaster. Instruct the patient to press the needles 50 times on each point, three times daily: morning, afternoon and evening. With each pressing, the patient should close their eyes and after pressing the ear point, focus their visual attention on a far subject for 10 minutes. After five days, change the needles and the plaster. Ten treatments constitute one course and it is important to rest one week between courses (two courses is usually sufficient).

Result

500 cases were treated with the above method: 48 cases completely resolved; 146 cases significantly improved; 218 cases slightly improved; and 88 cases had no change. The total efficacy rate was 82%. Note: *Complete resolution* refers to visual improvement above 1.0; *significantly improved* refers to visual improvement above 0.8; and *slightly improved* indicates visual improvement above 0.6.

Case

Li xx, male, 11 year-old student: Presented with a decrease in vision for the past year. The vision in his right eye tested at 0.1 and the vision in his left eye tested at 0.5. After one course of the above treatment method, both of Li's eyes tested at 1.5. After a second course of treatment, his eyes were tested again six months later and had sustained at 1.5.

Discussion

This method is most suitable for patients younger than 18 years old, and is most successful in patients less than 12 years old.

5.5 Deafness

Deafness, or sensory-neural hearing loss, can occur abruptly and for unknown reasons. Main clinical manifestations include a sudden and profound reduction (or elimination) of hearing, accompanied by tinnitus and dizziness. Such presentations have a tendency to resolve as spontaneously as they presented. The disorder is usually unilateral and occurs more often in females and mostly in the middle-aged.

Point

Tinggong (SI 19)

Location

Tinggong (SI 19) is located anterior to the tragus and posterior to the condyloid process of the mandible, in the depression formed when the mouth is open.

Method

Acupuncture is used. Have the patient in a seated position with their mouth open as wide as possible. Insert 1.5 cun needles perpendicularly to a depth of about 1.0 cun into each point, angling the needle toward the opposite ear. Once the needles are in place, the patient may close their mouth. Retain the needles for 30 minutes. During this time, instruct the patient to pinch their nose closed with their thumb and forefinger, and breathe in through their mouth and attempt to force the air out of their ears. For optimum results, some sound can be heard escaping from the ear. One course includes ten treatments.

Result

Acute cases can yield positive results within one or two treatments. Chronic cases usually require more than ten treatments for best results.

Case

Lu xx, male, 40 year-old farmer: Presented in seemingly good health, with a tendency for anxiety and a large consumption of alcohol. When angered, he notes feeling a headache, dizziness and a sudden loss of hearing. His traditional Chinese medicine diagnosis was deafness and anxiety from hyperactivity of liver yang. After five treatments by the above method, his symptoms and tendencies completely resolved.

Discussion

This method is suitable for anxiety-induced deafness, without any organic problems.

5.6 Tinnitus

Tinnitus is characterized by a subjective awareness of ringing in the ears, which cannot be alleviated by pressure or other measure. Tinnitus may also be accompanied by irritability or anger, dizziness, soreness and aching of the lower back, seminal emission, or excessive leukorrhea. When due to deficiency, the ringing may be further aggravated by overwork.

Point

Yemen (SJ 2)

Location

Yemen (SJ 2) is located in the depression proximal to the margin of the web between the ring and small fingers when the fingers are clenched into a fist, at the junction of the red and white skin.

Method

Acupuncture is used. Insert a 1cun needle horizontally and towards the metacarpal bone into each point, about 1cun deep. Rotate the needles about 10 times, until the patient can feel a Qi sensation travel up the arm. Retain the needles for 30~60 minutes. Manipulate the needles again every 10 minutes while the patient simultaneously pinches their nose closed and breathes in through the mouth and forces the air out of their ears. The treatment is most effective when some sound can be heard escaping from the ear. One course equals ten treatments.

Result

204 cases were treated with this method: 80 cases completely resolved; 52 cases significantly improved; 52 cases slightly improved; and 20 cases showed no change. The total efficacy rate was 91%.

Case

Wu xx, female, 25 years old: Presented with subjective ringing in her ears for more than one month, without any known cause. She went to a western Ear-Nose-Throat doctor, but received no relief. Her traditional Chinese medicine diagnosis was tinnitus due to Sanjiao Fire. While the acupuncturist was manipulating the needles during the treatment, the patient noted feeling a hot sensation in her ear. After the treatment, the ringing in her ears decreased and her hearing had improved. After four more treatments, the tinnitus had resolved.

5.7 Meniere's disease

The clinical characteristics of Meniere's disease included paroxysmal dizziness, fluctuating deafness, tinnitus and a feeling of fullness in the ear. It belongs to the category of "xuan yun" (dizziness) in traditional Chinese medicine.

Point

Baihui (DU 20)

Location

Baihui (DU 20) is located on the midline of the head, 5 cun directly above the midpoint of the anterior hairline, approximately on the midpoint of the line connecting the apexes of both ears.

Method

Direct moxibustion (non-scarring) is used. Have the patient seated in a chair and trim the hair 1cm circumference around the point. Apply burn-cream or vaseline onto the point. Use about 50 small moxa cones, each the size of a grain of rice. To complete, the treatment will take about one hour, after which a scab will form and fall away within a month. One treatment should be sufficient.

Result

177 cases were treated with this method: 156 cases completely resolved; 19 cases improved; and two cases had no effect. The total efficacy rate of this treatment was 98.88%.

Case

Zhou xx, male, 60 year-old worker: Presented with sudden onset of dizziness, tinnitus and vomiting. The traditional Chinese medicine diagnosis was Meniere's disease due to deficiency of Qi and blood. After one treatment using the above method, he felt better. At a five-year follow-up the symptoms had not recurred.

Discussion

Meniere's disease is usually due to deficiency of Qi and blood, or deficiency of kidney essence. The point Baihui (DU 20) has a special function to strengthen the Yin and Yang, and to nourish Qi, blood, and kidney essence.

5.8 Rhinitis

The term "Rhinitis" includes such presentations as acute rhinitis, chronic rhinitis, atrophic rhinitis, and allergic rhinitis. Acute rhinitis is a sudden infectious inflammation of the nasal mucosa. The clinical features include a burning feeling in the nose, nasal obstruction, sneezing, rhinorrhea, headache and fever. Chronic rhinitis refers to long-term inflammatory change of the nasal mucosa, mainly due to the protraction of acute rhinitis. The main clinical symptom is nasal obstruction. Atrophic rhinitis is a chronic change of the nasal mucosa and nasal cavity, often presenting with superficial crusts. Allergic rhinitis occurs when an allergic substance acts on the mucous membranes of the nasal cavity causing itching in the nose, sneezing, watery nasal discharge and congestion.

Point

Yingxiang (LI 20)

Location

Yingxiang (LI 20) is located in the naso-labial groove, at the level of the midpoint of the lateral border of ala nasi.

Method

Electric acupuncture is used. Locate the points bi-laterally. Insert 1.0 cun needles horizontally and angled toward the bridge to a depth of 0.8 cun. Rotate both needles at the same time, until a Qi sensation can be felt around the entire nose. Place an electrical device on the tip of the needles for 30 minutes, using the strongest continuous wave the patient can bear. Apply once daily, and ten sessions constitutes one treatment course.

Result

360 cases with many variations of rhinitis were treated with the above method: 176 cases (49%) significantly improved; 142 cases (39%) slightly improved; and 42 cases (12%) had no change. The efficacy rate improved after 3-5 treatments. The maximum number of treatments any of the participating patients received was twenty, the minimum was eight and the average number of treatments received was thirteen.

Case

Cai xx, female, 36 year-old worker: Presented with itching and a runny nose for the past three years. Her symptoms worsened in the winter and she had taken a lot of medicine (both Western and Chinese), without result. After one treatment with electric acupuncture, her nasal congestion had noticeably decreased. All other symptoms had ceased with the completion of one course of treatment.

Discussion

This method is suitable for any kind of rhinitis. In general, it is most effective in cases of chronic rhinitis.

5.9 Epistaxis

Epistaxis (or, nosebleed) is a common clinical symptom, and can be caused by a variety of reasons. Most often, the bleeding is seen in Kiesselbach's (the area at the naso-pharyngeal plexus at the end of the inferior nasal meatus). In traditional Chinese medicine, this condition is called "bi nu" (nose bleed), "bi hong" (flood-like nose bleed), and "hong han" (red sweat) - all referring to epistaxis.

Point

Shangxing (DU 23)

Location

Shangxing (DU 23) is located 1cun directly above the midpoint of the anterior hairline.

Method

Acupuncture is used. Insert a 2.0cun needle horizontally towards Baihui (DU 20) to a depth of 1.5cun. Manipulate the needle by rotating it for three minutes, every 10 minutes. Retain the needle for a total of 30 minutes. The bleeding should stop within the first few minutes of treatment.

Result

17 cases were treated with this method: 16 cases (95.3%) resolved after the first session and found immediate relief within an average of 1.5 minutes of needle insertion; and one case had no change and did not repeat treatment.

Case

Liu xx, male, 35 year-old, teacher, he presented with a sudden nosebleed that would not stop. He had tried several methods, including cotton, medicine, herbs and had no result. After three minutes of the above acupuncture treatment, the nosebleed had stopped. The needles were retained for 10 minutes and there was no further bleeding after 30 minutes of observation.

5.10 Acute Tonsillitis

Acute tonsillitis is a sudden, nonspecific inflammation of the palatal tonsils. Clinical features include fever, headache, a sore throat that is aggravated upon swallowing, and red, swollen palatal tonsils.

Point

Shaoshang (LU 11)

Location

Shaoshang (LU 11) is located on the radial side of the thumbnail, about 0.1 cun posterior to the corner of the nail.

Method

Three-edge needle therapy is used. Locate Shaoshang (LU11) on the affected side of the pain (if both sides are painful then use the points bilaterally). Insert a three-edged needle 0.1cun into the point(s), after sterilizing the area. Apply pressure and wipe away any blood with an alcohol soaked cotton ball. Repeat the process until the patient has bled a total of three times. After the last time, press the area with a dry cotton ball to stop the bleeding. Repeat once daily; 3-5 treatments is usually enough.

Result

164 cases were treated with this method: 108 cases (65.8%) completely resolved within 3-5 treatments; 38 cases (23.2%) improved with in 6-7 treatments; and 18 cases (11%) had no effect after eight treatments.

Case

Liu xx, male, 12 year-old student: Presented with tonsillitis after catching a common cold. Other symptoms included fever (his temperature was 38°C), chills, throat pain, and he had difficulty eating and drinking. The local area of his throat was swollen and red and the mandibular lymph nodes on either side of his neck were enlarged. Liu's tongue was red with yellow coating and his pulse was superficial and rapid. After the first treatment, his pain and fever decreased. Within four bilateral treatments, the tonsillitis was completely cured.

Discussion

1. Shaoshang (LU 11) belongs to the lung meridian and is on a specific branch of the lung meridian that passes through the throat. Shaoshang (LU 11) is therefore able to clear heat from both the lung meridian and the throat.

2. It is commonly thought that the more blood that is released, the more effective the treatment.

5.11 Plum-Pit Qi of the Throat

Plum-Pit Qi refers to the subjective feeling of a foreign body lodged in the throat, as if by the pit of a plum. Main characteristics include a constant dry cough, itching, an inability to expectorate anything and repeated swallowing without relief. A sensation of fullness of the chest and hypochondriac region, and emotional depression may also accompany Plum-Pit Qi. Adult females most often present with this condition. According to western medicine, this presentation is included in neurosis, globus hystericus, or plum-pit syndrome.

Point

Tiantu (RN 22)

Location

Tiantu (RN 22) is located in the center of the suprasternal fossa.

Method

Acupuncture is used. Have the patient in a seated position with their head tilted back. Insert a 2.0 cun needle perpendicularly to a depth of 0.2 cun, then change the direction to horizontal and facing downward. Continue to insert obliquely to a depth of 1.5 cun, until the patient can feel a Qi sensation inside the throat and chest. At that point, remove the needle.

Result

28 cases were treated with this method: 23 cases resolved after one treatment; two cases resolved after three treatments; and three cases had no change after three treatments.

Case

Liang xx, female, 48 years old: Presented with a sensation of something in her throat that she could not expel for the past three years. When she went to her western doctor for an evaluation, there was nothing abnormal. Her traditional Chinese medicine diagnosis was Qi stagnation. After one acupuncture treatment by the above method, her symptoms resolved.

Discussion

This point is known as the *'gate of the breath'* and can regulate the breath and balance the Qi of the organs. Because Plum-Pit Qi is caused by the stagnation of Qi, Tiantu (RN 22) can effectively resolve the problem.

5.12 Oral Ulcerations

This condition refers to scattered, superficial, small ulcerations in the mucous membrane of the mouth. Such ulcerations may come in either single or multiple degrees, and belong to the category of "kou gan" or "kou chuang," in traditional Chinese medicine (both referring to "ulcer of the mouth").

Point

Shenque (RN 8)

Location

Shenque (RN 8) is located on the middle of the abdomen and at the center of the umbilicus.

Method

Moxibustion is used. Ignite a Moxa stick and place it about 2.0 cm above the umbilicus. Move in a circular motion and in a sparrow-pecking motion for 10 minutes, or until the local area is red. Repeat once daily.

Result

104 cases were treated with this method: 58 cases completely resolved after 1-2 treatments; 30 cases completely resolved after three treatments; 12 cases did not change after three treatments times; and four cases did not stay for treatment.

Case

Zhou xx, female, 61 year-old farmer: Presented with ulcerative sores around her lips, severe pain, and an inability to eat or drink. After one treatment of moxibustion, her pain had decreased. After two treatments, the pain and the ulcerative areas decreased even further. Complete resolution was achieved after five treatments.

5. 13 TMJ Syndrome

TMJ (Temporal-Mandibular Joint) syndrome refers to pain, distension and soreness of the temporal-mandibular joint. There is often limited ability to open the mouth and a clicking sound produced upon movement of the jaw in TMJ Syndrome. These symptoms may also be accompanied by dizziness or tinnitus.

Point

Xiaguan (ST 7)

Location

Xiaguan (ST 7) is located anterior to the ear, on the face and in the depression between the zygomatic arch and the mandibular notch.

Method

Acupuncture is used. Insert a 1cun needle into each point bilaterally to a depth of 0.8cun deep. Manipulate the needles by lifting and thrusting until the patient can feel a Qi sensation in the whole local area. Retain the needles for 15 minutes and repeat the treatment once daily. One course is equal to 15 treatments.

Result

33 cases were treated with this method: 25 cases completely resolved; 13 cases improved; and five cases had no change.

Case

Qian xx, male, 25 years old: Presented with joint pain on the right side of his jaw for the past two weeks. When he opened his mouth, you could hear a sound come from the joint. He also had limited movement of his mouth, difficulty eating, and the pain was worse with palpation. Treatment with the above method completely resolved his symptoms within eight sessions.

5.14 Smoking Cessation

In this treatment approach, acupuncture is used to help patients to dislike the smell of cigarette smoke in order to achieve smoking cessation.

Point

Tim Mee (Experiential Point)

Location

Tim Mee (experiential point) is located in the depression midway between the two points Yangxi (LI 5) and Lieque (LU 7) (See Fig. 5-3).

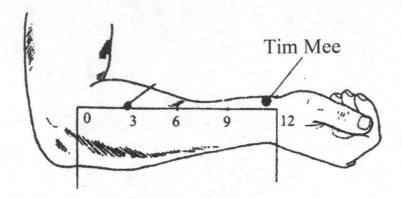

Fig. 5-3 Tim Mee (Experiential Point)

Method

Intradermal (embedding) therapy is used. Apply small intradermal needles bilaterally onto the points and cover each with a plaster. When the patient has an urge to smoke, instruct them to press the needle 20 times at each point. While applying pressure, a sweet sensation might be tasted under the tongue (which is normal). Leave the needles and plasters on for three days, then change.

Result

535 cases were treated with this method: 75% of the cases succeeded in quitting smoking after one treatment; 9% of the remaining cases succeeded after two treatments; and 16% of the remaining cases did not succeed in quitting smoking.

Case

Lai xx, male 18 year-old worker: Presented with a smoking habit of 30 cigarettes daily for the past three years. In addition, he felt dizziness, nausea, tastelessness in the mouth, and presented with a pale face. Lai decreased his cigarette smoking to 10 a day after one treatment and after two more treatments, he had ceased smoking completely.

Discussion

The most effective results with this therapy occur when the patient has a sincere desire to stop and/or control the amount of cigarettes they smoke. In cases where there is no desire to stop smoking, the effects will be minimal to none at all.

5.15 Dispelling the Effects of Alcohol

This refers to alleviating the feelings of nausea, vomiting, lethargy or coma accompanied by an over-consumption of alcohol.

Point

Suliao (DU 25)

Location

Suliao (DU 25) is located on the tip of the nose.

Method

Acupuncture is used. Insert a 0.5 cun needle perpendicularly into the point at a depth of 0.2cun. Stimulate the needle with a reducing method and retain for 30 minutes. Every five minutes manipulate the needle until the person wakes up or symptoms resolve.

Result

This method is effective in reviving an unconscious person due to consuming too much alcohol.

Case

An alcoholic patient loses consciousness and the ability to speak or control their movement. After using this method of treatment for 10 minutes, his consciousness was restored.

5.16 Weight Loss

Obesity refers to the excessive accumulation of fat in the subcutaneous or other body tissues by at least 15-20% over the normal weight. Clinically, obesity can be divided into simple and secondary types. The former is mainly due to over eating of greasy or sweet food, resulting in the accumulation of fat in the body. Such patients do not present with endocrine dysfunction. Secondary obesity results from hypothalamic pituitary lesions leading to an over-secretion of hydrocortisone, causing the body to store excess fat.

Point

Guanyuan (RN 4)

Location

Guanyuan (RN 4) is located on the anterior midline, 3cun below the umbilicus.

Method

Acupressure is used. Self-application of acupressure is done while the patient is lying in a supine position. Have the patient press and rotate the point in a circular motion for 30 minutes once daily. Repeat for 25 days or more, as needed.

Result

44 cases were treated with this method: 35 cases lost from 1-5 kg after 25 days of treatment; and nine cases did not lose any weight.

Case

Zhang xx, male, 42 year-old worker: Presented with clinical obesity for the past four years, weighing 70 kg (154 lbs) and 160cm (5.2 ft) tall. After treating himself with the above method, he lost 5 kg within 25 days.

Discussion

The patient's cooperation is required. It is recommended that the patient alter their diet to include primarily vegetables, a little red meat, chicken, and very little sugar. In addition, the patient should do half an hour to an hour of exercise every day.

About the Author

Dr. Decheng Chen is a Licensed Acupuncturist (L.Ac.), with a Ph.D. in Acupuncture and Traditional Chinese Medicine (TCM). He also holds a Traditional Medical Degree in China. In the United States, he holds an acupuncture license in New York, New Jersey and California. Currently, he practices in New York City. Dr. Chen was also a professor at the New York college of Traditional Chinese Medicine.

Dr. Decheng Chen graduated and received his Bachelor and Masters degrees from Changchun University of TCM in China and his Ph.D from Nanjing University of TCM in China. He studied under the famous professor, Dr. Qiu Maoliang, and learned acupuncture from him for three years. Before coming to the United States, he worked as a professor in The Acupuncture Hospital of China Academy of Chinese Medical Science in Beijing. He has had more than 20 years of clinical and teaching experience in China, Russia, Egypt, Dubai, U.A.E. and the United States.

Some of his published works include: (1) *Simplified Review for National Examinations in Acupuncture and Clean Needle Technique, 2003.* (2) *The Chinese Single Point Acupuncture and Moxibustion.* (3) *The Chinese Double Points Acupuncture and Moxibustion.* (4) *The Chinese Multiple Points Acupuncture and Moxibustion.* (5) *The Chinese Acupuncture and Moxibustion for Beauty and Anti-aging.* (6) *Hand and Foot Therapy of Acupuncture and Moxibustion.* In all, he has published 12 books, a DVD, more than 80 articles on Chinese Medicine, and has received numerous honors and recognitions for his work.

He has undertaken the following research: (1) A study on Single Point Therapy. (2) Clinical and Experimental Studies in the Treatment of Diabetes Mellitus with Acupuncture. (3) Clinical and Experimental Studies of Chronic Atrophic Gastritis Treated with Acupuncture and Moxibustion. All of them received much recognition and awards from the government in china.

Contact Information:

Add: 1 west 34th Street Suite 903
New York, NY 10001
Tel: 212-564-3324
Fax: 212-564-3732
Email: dechengchen2000@yahoo.com
Web: www.go2acupuncture.com

The Author's Publishing List

Author's Bibliography

1. *The Clinical Application of Double-Point Acupuncture and Moxibustion Therapy* (English version/ 266 pages). Trafford Publishing, 2007.

2. *Simplified Review for National Examinations in Acupuncture and Clean Needle Technique* (English version/ 360 pages). Trafford Publishing, 2003.

3. *Complete Collection of Chinese Acupuncture and Moxibustion for Cosmetic and Anti-aging* (Chinese version / 576 pages). China Traditional Chinese Medicine Publish If House, China. 2002

4. *100 Diseases Treated by Single Point of Acupuncture and Moxibustion* (English version/ 200 pages). Foreign Languages Press, Beijing, China, 2001.

5. *Chronic Gastritis* (Chinese version / 117 pages). China Traditional Chinese Medicine Publish House, China, 2000.

6. *Hand and foot Acupuncture Therapy* (Chinese version / 466 pages). Shanghai Science and Technology Publish House, China.2000

7. *The Chinese Double Points Acupuncture and Moxibustion* (Chinese version / 576 pages). Jilin Science and Technology Publish House, China, 1998.

8. *The Chinese Multiple Points Acupuncture and Moxibustion.* (Chinese version / 996 pages), Gueizhou Science and Technology Publish House, China, 1995

9. *Complete Collection of Traditional Therapy* (Chinese version / 1242 pages). Changchun Publish House, China, 1995.

10. *The Chinese Single Point Acupuncture and Moxibustion* (Old Chinese version/ 1400 pages). Taiwan Fuwen Publish Stock Limited Company, China.1995.

11. ***Complete Collection Micro-Acupuncture Therapy*** (Chinese version / 377 pages). Science and Technology Publish Company, China, 1995.

12. ***The Chinese Single Point Acupuncture and Moxibustion*** (Chinese version/ 860 pages). Jilin Science and Technology Publish House, China, 1993.

Author's Discography

1. ***The Chinese Single Point Acupuncture and Moxibustion.*** (English version/ 96 minutes). 2003

2. ***The Chinese Single Point therapy of Acupuncture and Moxibustion.*** (Chinese version/ 94 minutes). 1998

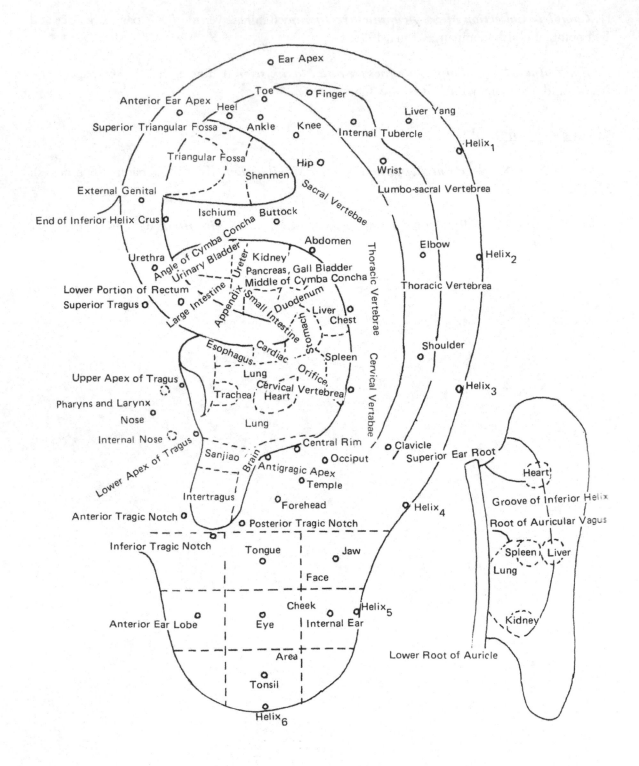

Auricular point pictures